OWN YOUR HEALTH

The Best of Alternative & Conventional Medicine

Pain

BACK PAIN, ARTHRITIS, MIGRAINES,
JOINT PAIN AND MORE

ADAM PERLMAN, M.D., MPH

EXECUTIVE DIRECTOR
INSTITUTE FOR COMPLEMENTARY AND ALTERNATIVE MEDICINE
UNIVERSITY OF MEDICINE AND DENTISTRY OF NEW JERSEY

AND ROANNE WEISMAN

Health Communications, Inc.
Deerfield Beach, Florida

www.hcibooks.com

This book is not intended to be a substitute for the advice and/or medical care of the reader's physician. The reader should consult with a physician in all matters related to his or her health.

Library of Congress Cataloging-in-Publication Data available from the Library of Congress

© 2006 Adam Perlman and Roanne Weisman
ISBN-13: 978-0-7573-0492-7
ISBN-10: 0-7573-0492-3

Publisher: Health Communications, Inc.
            3201 S.W. 15th Street
            Deerfield Beach, FL 33442–8190

Cover and inside book design by Lawna Patterson Oldfield
Cover photos ©Artville, ©Shutterstock
Inside book formatting Dawn Von Strolley Grove

CONTENTS

Preface by Roanne Weisman v
Introduction ix

1 Acute Pain: When to Get Help 1
2 Taking Control of Chronic Pain 15
3 Integrative Medicine for Chronic Pain:
   The Best Tools from Conventional
   and Alternative Medicine 31
   Osteoarthritis 36
4 The Biopsychosocial Approach:
   Treating More Than Pain 45
   Abdominal Pain 50
5 Biofeedback and Hypnotherapy for Pain 65
6 Diet: The Relationship Between Food
   and Pain 77
7 Acupuncture and Traditional Chinese
   Medicine: Restoring the Flow 87
   Fibromyalgia 95
8 The Alexander Technique: Using the Mind
   to Free the Body from Pain 101

 9 **Cranial Osteopathy and Craniosacral Therapy:
   Movement Is All** 109
10 **Chiropractic**..119
   Lower Back and Pelvic Pain................................123
11 **Ayurvedic Medicine** 127
   Headache and Migraine.......................................135
12 **Massage Therapy**...139
13 **The Trager® Approach: Easing Mind
   and Body** 151
14 **Meditation: Don't Miss a Moment
   of Your Life** 157

Resources..165
Notes 172

PREFACE

To me, "owning my health" means taking as much responsibility as possible for what goes on in my body. It is the opposite of feeling like a helpless victim of pain, disease or disability. It also means working in a collaborative partnership with my doctor to find the best ways to prevent and treat disease from *all* worlds of medicine: alternative and complementary as well as conventional.

Here is how I learned to "own my health": In 1995 I woke up from heart valve surgery with the left side of my body paralyzed from a stroke. A tiny piece of tissue had broken away from the valve, traveled through blood vessels and lodged in my brain, blocking the flow of blood with its essential supply of oxygen to the neurons that controlled movement on my left side.

If I had obediently followed the prescribed role of stroke patient in the world of conventional medicine, I would be dependent on adaptive devices and other people for many of the activities of daily life.

Instead, I have recovered completely and am back to my life as a medical journalist, wife and mother.

I quickly learned that while the advances of modern medicine can save your life, the conventional medical system—along with the insurers who pay for it—is not set up for true healing. The goal of the system was to get me to a minimal level of functioning, out of the hospital or rehabilitation facility, and back home. What happened after that was up to me.

As a patient, it often feels as if the conventional health care system wants us to accept and "adapt" to our health problems—whether we are recovering from a heart attack or stroke or suffering from chronic illness or pain. We often feel as if we are being treated as collections of body parts to be "fixed" with pills or adaptive devices, rather than as whole people with emotions, relationships, minds and spirits.

By contrast, "integrative medicine," which is the philosophy of this *Own Your Health* book series, encourages people to combine complementary and alternative medicine (often called "CAM") with conventional medicine to find true healing of body, mind and spirit—to achieve wholeness.

When you are in chronic pain, you often feel particularly alone in the world of conventional medicine. The cause of chronic pain is often difficult to diagnose and treat, and as Dr. Adam

Perlman notes in the Introduction, pain can cause problems in every area of your life.

Going outside of the conventional medical system can be a tough thing for many of us, but with Dr. Perlman's guidance, you will learn about many effective options for controlling and managing pain. When I looked for ways to expand my own healing options, I found treatments that helped me both recover movement and reduce pain. These included acupuncture and tai chi from the ancient system of Traditional Chinese Medicine; yoga from the equally ancient Indian Ayurvedic system of medicine; the Alexander Technique—a powerful system of movement education that teaches you to use your body with less effort and reduced pain; craniosacral therapy; and various forms of bodywork and massage. As you will see in this book, these and many other healing methods—such as herbal medicine—are particularly effective for reducing chronic pain.

I am grateful that Dr. Perlman, executive director of the Institute for Complementary and Alternative Medicine at the University of Medicine and Dentistry of New Jersey, is the co-author of this book. Dr. Perlman's research and clinical practice focus on general wellness, fibromyalgia, chronic pain and cancer. In addition, Dr. Perlman is director of Integrative Medicine for the Saint Barnabas Health Care System and medical director for the Carol and Morton Siegler Center for Integrative Medicine in New Jersey, where he has been recognized by his peers with the Excellence in Caring award.

Dr. Perlman and I also appreciate the valuable advice contributed by three other health professionals: Gary L. Golberg, Ph.D., who specializes in health psychology and mind/body medicine; Dale Bellisfield, R.N., A.H.G., a certified herbalist who combines herbal medicine, diet, supplements and lifestyle in the treatment of many chronic conditions, including pain; and certified hypnotherapist Julietta Appleton. And finally, we wish to thank Brian Berman, M.D., director of integrative medicine at the University of Maryland, for his expertise in the treatment of pain and for sharing information about his recent, significant research on the use of acupuncture in the treatment of low back pain as well as for osteoarthritis of the knee.

We hope that this book will help you achieve healing and wholeness and manage your pain by "owning your health."

—*Roanne Weisman*

INTRODUCTION

Make no mistake, pain is a warning that something is wrong. If you are in pain, and your doctor cannot determine the physical cause, no one should tell you "it is all in your mind." Pain is experienced mentally as well as physically; therefore, if you are feeling pain, it is real. Pain affects not only a person's ability to function physically, it may also affect functioning on an emotional and spiritual level. Your quality of life may be diminished; you may feel as if you have to put your dreams and goals on hold; you might have lost the connection with yourself that allows you to understand what gives your life meaning and purpose; and your relationships with others may be damaged.

In this book, we will give you suggestions—backed up by published research—for combining alternative and conventional treatments to reduce both the causes of your pain and the symptoms you are feeling. These suggestions will give you more "tools for your tool belt," to understand and manage your pain. But unlike the conventional medical approach, we will also address the spiritual and emotional costs of pain.

This perspective of looking at the whole person and considering issues of mind, body and spirit is the basis of "integrative medicine." As an integrative physician, I look at my patients as whole people, not merely collections of ailing body parts to be fixed. I want to help my patients—and you—achieve *healing* in body, mind and spirit. Even when pain cannot be completely eliminated, there are always ways you can be supported so that the effect pain is having on your quality of life is diminished and you feel a greater sense of control.

In the world of integrative medicine, "healing" is very different from "curing." It means that you are connected with your deepest self and experience the intimate interaction between your body, mind and spirit in order to feel whole. It means that you can draw upon the tools of conventional medicine and combine them with the wisdom of many alternative treatments, some of which are thousands of years old.

Massage therapy, for example, has been a health practice of most ancient cultures, including China, India, Persia, Arabia and Greece. Hippocrates used massage to treat sprains and dislocations, Aristotle treated exhaustion by massaging the body with oil and water, and oil massage was used in Sparta and Athens in preparation for vigorous exercise. Descriptions of tui na (a form of massage) and acupressure, both from the system of Traditional Chinese Medicine, appeared in the pages of *The Yellow Emperor's Classic of Medicine*, written 2,500 years ago and believed to be the first book of Chinese medicine. Indian Ayurvedic practices date back to the fifth century BC. The recent revival of infant massage in this country has been patterned on the ancient practice of Indian baby massage.[1] You will learn about all of these methods—as well as several other ways of treating pain—in this book.

The Integrative Approach to Pain: What Does It Mean to Own Your Health?

Your body is designed to heal itself and find the balance of health that is right for you. Tapping into this healing ability is especially important when you are in chronic pain. We all have the innate capacity to restore balance, repair damaged cells and recover from illness. Problems arise when these natural healing abilities are blocked, either by stress, poor diet or a lifestyle that demands too much of us. Conventional medicine is good at curing certain diseases and treating the symptoms of illness and injury. At times, the conventional medical approach is clearly the right answer. However, conventional medicine is less effective at helping to stimulate our own natural healing abilities and less focused on treating the whole person.

Integrative medicine, on the other hand, recognizes that we are more than the cells, molecules and atoms that make up our bodies. We all have something else—something that won't show up on an x-ray or CT scan. We can call this our life force, "Qi" (pronounced "chi"), spirit, energy or many other names. But whatever we call it, it is this intangible "energy" that heals. It empowers our immune systems so that our bodies can repair damage from the stress, bacteria, viruses, pollution, injuries and other onslaughts that most of us deal with every day. The Consortium for Academic Health Centers for Integrative Medicine recently defined integrative medicine as "the practice of medicine that reaffirms the importance of relationship between practitioner and patient, focuses on the whole person, is informed by evidence, and makes use of all appropriate therapeutic approaches to achieve optimal health and healing."

The suggestions in this book are designed to help you work with your health care provider—using integrative medicine—to find the resilience that will help you free your body of pain.

This book is divided into chapters on different methods of treating pain using both conventional and alternative medicine. For each of these methods, we have described the treatment, "introduced" you to a practitioner, and provided evidence of its effectiveness (or lack thereof) for particular ailments. In addition, we have included sections describing the best integrative treatments for the most common chronic pain conditions. This information is designed to help you work in partnership with your doctor to combine conventional and alternative treatments that reduce your particular pain.

The Importance of "Owning Your Health" When You Are in Pain

"Your health is in your hands," says Ester R. Shapiro, Ph.D. "Although you may not have control of the course of an illness, how you respond to that illness—drawing on the support of family, community, your own beliefs and spiritual values—can help you heal." A psychologist, researcher, writer and teacher, Shapiro notes that only approximately 10 percent of health outcomes are produced by any contact with the health system. As much as 90 percent are due to your lifestyle, economic resources, social support, and a sense of power in determining the course and condition of your life and the lives of your family and community. Research shows that people who feel a sense of control—of ownership—of their health do better clinically than those who feel they are helpless victims of their illness.

Shapiro's writing and work focus on the way in which people and their families deal with extraordinary life challenges, including pain, illness and death by achieving resilience and wholeness.[2] "How do people succeed in overcoming adversity?" she asks. "What resources in their environment—family, religion, culture and community—combine with their own personal resources to build *resilience*? Resilient people know how to look for things that might help them recover from illness, while others might feel overwhelmed and defeated."[3]

Several stories in this book illustrate how patients with severe, unrelenting pain were able to use integrative medicine to achieve this "wholeness." They found ways to heal their bodies, minds and spirits and to reduce or eliminate their pain. In this book, we do not restrict ourselves to only one approach to pain. We draw on the science of conventional medicine as well as effective treatments from complementary and alternative medicine to give you the best of *all* worlds.

—*Adam Perlman, M.D., MPH, FACP*

1

ACUTE PAIN:
WHEN TO GET HELP

The biggest mistake that people make is to treat pain on their own without knowing the cause. This can be dangerous or even life-threatening. If, for example, you have a pain in your belly, and you take an over-the-counter pain medicine, you might be covering up the symptoms of appendicitis, which often requires immediate surgery. So the first step when you are in pain is to determine what is causing it. The next step is to decide what to do about it. This book will give you the information and the tools to do both. You will learn when to call the doctor, when to take medicine, when to go to the emergency room, and—if it is appropriate—when to use lifestyle modifications and alternative treatments that are the most effective for your pain.

There are two kinds of pain: acute and chronic. Acute pain usually comes on suddenly and has an obvious cause: a broken bone, an internal infection, a pulled muscle, a burn. This kind of pain usually requires conventional medical treatment such as surgery or drugs. Sometimes, acute pain requires emergency treatment, and for this you need to contact your doctor, go to the emergency room of a hospital or call for an ambulance. This first chapter lists the kinds of acute pain for which you should seek medical help, either at your doctor's office or in an emergency room.

Chronic pain, by contrast, is something that may have an obvious cause, like arthritis, or it may persist even after an injury has healed. But for many people with chronic pain, the cause is not immediately clear. This kind of pain is a frequent and unwelcome companion: aches and pains in the back, neck, shoulders or joints come and go with irritating regularity, often interfering with activities and the enjoyment of life.

Chronic pain is the major focus of this book. Most pain, particularly as we get older, is not a sign of something serious like cancer, but is a manifestation of general wear and tear on the joints, muscles and tissue that makes up our bodies. You do not have to suffer with chronic pain; there are ways to become more comfortable.

Acute Pain: When to Seek Help

It is important not to ignore certain kinds of pain.

Sometimes pain can be an early warning sign of a potentially serious illness or a tumor. The rest of this chapter gives you guidelines for the kind of pain for which you should seek immediate medical help.

Acute pain (coming from an actual or potential injury) keeps us safe: jerking our hand away from a hot stove or boiling water will prevent a burn, for example. People without adequate pain sensations can seriously injure themselves without realizing it. Following is a summary of pain that needs immediate medical attention. But if something isn't mentioned here, and if you're not sure, always call your doctor.

If you or your family members experience any of the pain symptoms described in this chapter, do not ignore them, hoping that they will go away. Take action, either by calling your doctor or going to the emergency room of a hospital. As a general rule: ***Do not ignore pain that is so severe that it keeps you up at night or pain that is new and unexplained.***

Head and Neck

Headache

We will discuss chronic headaches, such as migraines, later in this book. However, if you experience an acute, sharp headache that lasts more than an hour and is associated with blurry vision, difficulty talking, or weakness in the arms or legs, get immediate medical help. These symptoms may indicate a **stroke** or a **brain aneurysm**. In either case, minutes may make the difference between life and death, permanent disability and recovery.

Severe, intense headache with fever, cold symptoms, neck stiffness and drowsiness in children or adults may be a symptom of **meningococcal meningitis**—a life-threatening condition. Sometimes these symptoms are associated with a pinpoint red rash on the neck or upper chest. Call your doctor or 911, or go to the emergency room immediately.

Chest and Upper Back

Chest Pain

Pain in your chest that feels progressive in its severity—like heartburn or a weight on your chest—or that radiates into your left jaw, neck or arm, should be considered the symptoms of a **heart attack** until proven otherwise. If you experience these symptoms, chew a couple of aspirin tablets, stay calm and have someone drive you to an emergency room or call 911. If you feel lightheaded, dizzy or short of breath, call 911 immediately and notify your doctor.

Acute Pain Radiating from the Neck or Back

Acute, severe pain in the arms and/or legs that radiates from the neck or back and which may be associated with numbness, tingling, stabbing, burning or weakness may be a symptom of a **herniated disk in the spine**. What may be confusing about these symptoms is that they may not radiate from the spine. They are sometimes localized around the elbow, knee or ankle and may be confused with symptoms coming from these joints.

Between the vertebrae of your spine are disks.

These disks are made up of a tough outer rim, like a tire, and a gummy center, and they act as cushions between the bony vertebrae of your spine. If the rim develops a defect and the center bulges out, the disk is said to be herniated. If this bulge compresses a nerve leading to the arm or leg, it causes radiating symptoms of pain. The most common place for a herniated disk is in the low back, where it can press on the nerves leading to the sciatic nerve, causing **sciatica**—with pain radiating down the back of the buttocks, the front or back of the thigh, or lower leg and into the foot. A herniated disk can happen suddenly as the result of a movement, or the pain can develop more insidiously and gradually.

If the pain is severe and is associated with weakness or loss of sensation, stumbling or tripping, contact your physician or have someone take you to the emergency room.

Severe Back Pain Associated with Belly Tenderness

Acute, severe, unrelenting pain down the middle of your back or in the low back that is associated with belly pain may be a symptom of an **aortic aneurysm.** This is a bulge in the main artery leading away from the heart. Sometimes this bulge causes a slight tear in the aortic wall. This is an emergency. If the artery ruptures, it can result in death. You are more at risk for an aortic aneurysm if you are male and middle-aged or older. You are also at risk if you are or have been a smoker, either male or female.

Belly and Low Back

Belly Pain

Pain in your belly, particularly when it is associated with nausea and/or vomiting and tenderness to touch, should be considered a symptom of a condition called **"acute abdomen."** If this condition is associated with tenderness:

- On the lower right side, it could be **appendicitis**.
- On the upper right side, it could be **gall bladder disease**.
- On the upper left side, it could be **stomach ulcer**.
- On the lower left side, it could be **diverticulitis** (a pouch on the outside of the wall of the intestine that could rupture and lead to infection; classic symptoms include fever, decreased appetite and diarrhea).

All of these conditions should receive immediate medical attention.

Pain Between the Chest and Low Back

Acute, severe back pain at the junction between the chest and the low back can be a symptom of a **kidney stone.** This kind of pain usually starts on one side and radiates down into the flank and groin area. Pain from a kidney stone comes in spasms and is usually associated with nausea and sometimes with vomiting, sweating and lightheadedness. You may or may not have pain when urinating or have blood in the urine.

If you have this kind of pain, it soon becomes apparent that you need to go the emergency room. The pain is agonizing. It will not let up and there is nothing you can do to relieve it on your own. You should not try to "wait it out," since the kidney stone may not pass out of your body without medical intervention. Your doctor can give you medication to help get rid of the stone more quickly.

These symptoms may also indicate a **herniated disk** or **sciatica.** (See "Acute Pain Radiating from the Neck or Back.")

Shoulder, Arm and Hand

Shoulder Pain

Pain in the shoulder is very commonly associated with arthritis or bursitis. But if you are unable to raise your arm from your side, you may have a **frozen shoulder**. This condition typically occurs after trauma to the shoulder and may be dramatically relieved by acupuncture. More commonly, however, the condition is effectively treated by supervised physical therapy. Massage is *not* a good idea for a frozen shoulder as it causes irritation and may make it worse.

Pain and Numbness in the Hand

If you wake at night with pain in your hand associated with numbness, particularly in the thumb, index and middle fingers, stand up and shake your hand. If this relieves the pain and numbness, you could have **carpal tunnel syndrome**. Although this condition is usually attributed to overuse and repetitive activities such as typing, it is also associated with some form of arthritis or diabetes. See a hand specialist if these symptoms interfere with your daily activities or regularly disturb your sleep.

Hips, Legs and Feet

Aching in Legs

An aching sensation down the front and outside of the lower leg below the knee that becomes more intense with fast walking or running is a symptom of **shin splints**. If it lasts after exercising and is bad enough to make you lie down and you are still in pain, it could also be a **stress fracture** in a lower leg bone. Both shin splints and stress fractures are common in long-distance runners, new army recruits and people who are out of shape.

Stress fractures can be dangerous if left untreated: They can develop into full-blown fractures in the hip, lower leg or foot, requiring orthopedic surgery that can take months to heal. Do not ignore them. See your doctor.

Aching and pain in the leg that does not go away after you stop walking or running may also be a symptom of **compartment syndrome**, which causes swelling in the muscle on the outside of the lower leg. It may also be a sign of poor circulation in the legs, called **intermittent claudication**. Compartment syndrome is an emergency, comparable to appendicitis, because if it is not immediately treated it can kill the muscle and cause permanent weakness in the foot. Claudication can be treated by your physician.

Pain and Swelling in the Foot

Pain in the base of the big toe that is severe and is associated with swelling and redness may be the first signs of **gout**. This is a form of arthritis in which uric acid crystals form in the joint and cause irritation. It can attack any joint and is usually attributed to eating rich foods. (Henry VIII is thought to have suffered from gout in his later years.) Most people who have gout, however, have an inherited weakness for the disorder. Gout needs to be diagnosed by a physician. If left untreated it can affect the kidneys.

Whole Body

Generalized Aches and Pains with Weakness, Sweatiness and Cold Symptoms

These symptoms are most commonly part of a flu syndrome, but if they are not, they could indicate a serious disorder called **polymyositis**. This is a rheumatologic disorder that affects muscles and tendons and requires treatment with steroids. Patients with polymyositis often delay seeking help from their doctors for several months. As soon as you begin to notice weakness in everyday activities, such as getting up from a chair, going up stairs or stepping up onto a curb, you should call your doctor.

Severe Joint or Bone Pain that Keeps You Up at Night

While arthritis pain is common, it is benign and can be treated. (See "Osteoarthritis" section.) However, severe pain in the bones and joints that gets worse and keeps you up at night should not be ignored. If this pain does not respond to rest or over-the-counter pain medication, call your doctor. This could be the symptom of an **infection**, **fracture** or **tumor**.

Painful, Burning, Linear Rash

If you have rash that is in a straight line, has a painful, burning sensation and makes your skin supersensitive to touch, you may have **shingles**. This is a viral infection of the sensory nerves that is highly contagious by touch and is caused by the same virus that causes chicken pox. Shingles can occur on the face or anywhere on the body, but it usually begins in the area of the spine and follows the pattern of the sensory nerves around one side of the body. Do not touch or scratch it and then rub your eyes because this virus can infect the eye and cause blindness. See a doctor as soon as you notice this rash. There is medication that can shorten the course and alleviate symptoms. The virus that causes shingles may lie dormant in the body for years, so it is hard to tell when exposure occurred.

Pain in Children

The general rule is: **Do not ignore pain in children.** Children typically do not complain of pain unless they have it. Under the age of two, children express pain through irritability or screaming if you touch or move a part of their bodies that hurts. Following a cold, infants can develop an infection in the bloodstream that can seep into any joint— especially the hip—that could damage the joint. In this situation, the baby will be irritable or scream if you touch or move the infected arm or a leg. Take the baby immediately to the emergency room. If the baby is rigid and stiff, especially in the neck, suspect **meningitis** and go immediately to the emergency room.

Older children complaining of belly pain may have **appendicitis**, which requires emergency treatment. Limping or joint pain might indicate an **injury** or **infection in the bone or joint**, which should be checked by your pediatrician. Neck stiffness may be a symptom of **meningitis**.

(For more information about children's illness, see *Own Your Health: Your Sick Child*, another book in the *Own Your Health* series.)

2

TAKING CONTROL OF
CHRONIC PAIN

Barbara thought that she was having another urinary tract infection. "I had had those before, and this pain felt similar," she says. "I assumed that, as usual, antibiotics would take care of it." But this time, the pain did not go away. In fact, it got worse. "During the next few days, it began to feel as if there were knives in my pelvis," says Barbara. "Over the course of the next several weeks, both my bladder and pelvis became so excruciatingly painful that I could no longer sit down. In fact, I spent the next seven months either standing up or lying down with a complex pillow arrangement. When I did manage to fall asleep, I could usually stay that way for a few hours. In the beginning, that was one of the only respites."

The pain began in 1999, when Barbara was in her mid-forties, and it remained the dominant force in her life for more than two years. Until then, she had lived a life free of any major health problems. Married for sixteen years with no children, she and her husband enjoyed being physically active. At the time the pain started, Barbara had a successful, home-based corporate consulting business. "Luckily, I was well positioned both to understand and manage the medical system," she says.

During the next two years, these analytic and management skills were to become Barbara's lifeline, as the conventional medical system initially failed to provide either diagnosis or treatment for the pain that was relentlessly taking over her life. Neurological and laboratory tests, pelvic exams and ultrasounds all came back negative. "The doctors seemed at a loss," says Barbara.

On her own, Barbara then embarked on a quest for relief in the world of alternative medicine. "I found that exercising helped," she says. "I also tried hot baths, meditation, a very slow form of meditative walking, as well as yoga. They helped somewhat, but most of the day was filled with pain, periods of which I can only describe as hellish." In addition to exercising, the only other time Barbara felt no pain was when she was standing at her raised computer table and writing. By this time, Barbara had stopped working. She could no longer drive or sit at meetings with clients. "So I wrote," she says. During the two years that followed, she kept a journal of her experiences. "One of the many life changes that came out of this pain was that I began to take my writing more seriously," says Barbara.

Despite continued testing, Barbara's primary care doctor and the various specialists could come up with no organic reason for the pain. "I was becoming desperate," says Barbara. "It was beginning to dawn on me that I had to give up the fantasy that some wise, all-knowing person would appear who would help me figure out what to do. Instead, I realized that I had to be the one to take control of my pain—to pursue a diagnosis and find ways to manage it. And this also meant that I had to be the integrator—the one who would bring together allopathic [conventional] and complementary/alternative medicine [also called 'CAM']. It was in my hands."

The Message of Chronic Pain: Remember You Are a Whole Person

Barbara's experience with pain is shared by millions of Americans. Here are some facts about chronic pain:

- Chronic pain is the nation's third greatest health care problem after heart disease and cancer.
- Thirty percent of the population in developed countries (which amounts to some 80 million people in this country alone) report some form of chronic pain during their lifetimes—and half of these people are either partially or totally disabled for periods of a few days to several months.
- Chronic pain costs the United States approximately $65 billion in health care and lost productivity every year.
- Seventy percent of people who seek out alternative or complementary therapies do so for pain-related problems.

The International Association for the Study of Pain defines pain as "an unpleasant sensory and emotional experience associated with actual or potential tissue damage, or described in terms of such damage. *It is always subjective in nature.*"

What does this mean, "always subjective in nature?" Brian Berman, M.D., director of integrative medicine at the University of Maryland, explains: "It means that whether or not we can find the physical cause of your pain, if you are feeling it, *it is real.* Our job as doctors is to find ways to stop it. We may try to stop it in the laboratory, by looking for ways to repair damaged nerve cells that are sending you pain messages. We may use some combination of drugs that decrease the intensity of pain messages that originate in the brain. We may also try to understand not only the physical experience of your pain, but also the mental, emotional and perhaps even the spiritual meaning of the pain."

Remember that the Own Your Health concept is based on the premise that people are more than just a collection of molecules that can be chemically adjusted to solve health problems. This is particularly true when we are in pain. Chronic persistent pain is a multidimensional problem. Like Barbara, you might be experiencing one or more of the following emotions:

- Fear
- Depression (because you can see no end in sight)
- Hopelessness
- Despair
- Isolation
- Feeling out of control, a victim of your body

If you are in this situation, you should look for a holistic, multidimensional solution, one that focuses not only on the physical cause of your pain, but also on you as a "whole person," with emotions, spirit and life-coping skills. (See "Resources" at the end of this book for guidelines to finding integrative pain care.)

"People are looking for relief from their pain, but they also want to be listened to and understood by their doctors," says Dr. Berman. "They do *not* want to be seen as a collection of defective molecules. They want a relationship with their physicians that is humane as well as healing."

Developing a Support System

While she was trying alternative methods, Barbara kept up with the conventional system, seeing a uro-gynecologist, as well as a specialist at a pain clinic who recommended neuropathic drugs. She also tried an antispasmodic medication. Nothing helped.

Throughout her decision-making process, Barbara used her primary care doctor as a kind of scientific sounding board. "He helped me weigh options analytically and also recommended further testing," she says. "Although he is not trained in complementary methods, he played a critical role in my care: He was compassionate, and he believed that I would recover. Often, he would call me from his car on his way home from work and just talk to me while I was lying on the couch, crying. It was so important for me just to have that connection with a healing person."

TIP

It is very important that you always include your primary care doctor in any exploration of alternative treatments. Do not try treatments, especially herbs, on your own, because they may have dangerous side effects or drug interactions that you may not be aware of.

After all of the tests and exams had ruled out any dangerous or acutely life-threatening conditions,

Barbara tried homeopathy, which uses minute amounts of medicine carefully tailored to each person's physical and emotional condition.

In addition to homeopathy, Barbara also tried acupuncture, chiropractic, craniosacral work and biofeedback. (See chapters that follow for a description of these treatments.) "But even with all of the specialists—both conventional and alternative—the pain medication, yoga and meditation, I still could not control the pain enough to function normally," says Barbara. "Finding a solution to a serious illness is hard under the best of circumstances, but when you are feeling physically devastated, it is nearly impossible, especially when you try to deal with the insurance bureaucracy!"

TIP

When you are struggling with chronic pain, it is important to develop a good support system, including family, friends and health professionals. Try to find people who take you seriously and who believe that you will get better.

Barbara found the support system she needed on her quest for relief: "Both the homeopath and my primary doctor would always return calls quickly, even over the weekend, and they, as well as my husband, kept telling me over and over again that things would get better. I felt like I was drowning, and their conviction gave me a life preserver to hang onto when I most needed it."

TIP

Try to distinguish between "curing" and "healing," especially when you are dealing with pain. Even if the pain cannot be eliminated, you can often control its intensity—and you can control your own perceptions of the meaning of the pain in your life.

Says Barbara: "I knew right from the beginning that the pain was appearing for a reason, and I needed to figure out that reason at this point in my life. I began to read everything I could find about illness as metaphor, to try to understand what my body was trying to tell me about my beliefs about myself, and about old wounds, both emotional and physical. Keeping a journal became one of my most important tools for self-understanding during that time, in addition to psychotherapy."

Finding the Right Doctor

Even as she searched for the meaning behind her pain, however, Barbara and her husband kept up their search for an effective treatment. They turned to the Internet and also began talking to everyone they could think of. Barbara was determined not to give up, to keep looking for specialists—either conventional or alternative—until she found those who could help her. "Desperate times call for desperate measures," says Barbara. "We cold-called specialists all over the country."

Finally, the answer came from a basketball game. "My brother plays basketball on Sundays with a group of other doctors, and he asked them if they knew of any good pain specialists in my city," says Barbara. "We got one highly recommended name. It took three months to get an appointment. I learned, by the way, to make a lot of appointments well in advance with specialists that you *think* you may want to see, because appointments can take months to get. I also learned how to work with secretaries to get notified of cancellations."

TIP

Make appointments early on with any specialists you think you might want to see, because it often takes months to get these appointments. Work with secretaries to get notified of cancellations.

In this case, the three-month wait was worth it. "This doctor was absolutely the right person for me to see," says Barbara. "He is a brilliant scientist and researcher, as well as a healer. He spent an hour with me on the first appointment; he calls me back and responds to e-mails." This doctor recommended a combination of drugs to manage the pain and decrease the intensity of pain messages that originate in the brain. Combinations had been tried before, says Barbara, "but this doctor had more experience with the medication interactions than the previous doctors. The drug 'cocktail' he put together helped tremendously." At the same time, Barbara began seeing an energy healer who did hands-on healing. "He was the only one who could actually bring my pain down quickly."

The pain "cocktail," acupuncture, energy work and Barbara's own inner psychological exploration combined to reduce and then eliminate her pain condition over a period of about four years. "It is hard to separate out the effect of each treatment," she says. "It was the *combination* that was powerful." Barbara is still followed by her pain specialist, although she has not needed medication for the pain condition for the past year. She continues to practice meditation, yoga and other mind/body activities, and does an hour and a half of aerobic exercise every day. She has also changed her career focus. She is back to consulting, but on a more limited basis, and is putting more energy into what she feels is her true vocation: writing. "The conventional and complementary track were two of my three sources of healing," she says. "The third was my own emotional healing, nurtured by my psychotherapist and my journal. The pain was the catalyst that helped me to rewrite the story of my life. I began to understand that the pain was my body's way of helping me be more in alignment with who I was meant to be."

✓ TAKE ACTION ✓

for Chronic Pain

Here are some ways to take control of chronic pain. Remember, you *should always consult first with your doctor* before beginning any new practice, treatment or medication.

- Keep a journal and a daily pain log, recording both the progression of the pain and what helps to reduce it.
- Write your own case history and update it regularly, describing the onset of pain, tests and results, therapies you have tried and their effectiveness. Send a copy to any new doctor or practitioner *before* your appointment. This saves you the time of endlessly repeating your story and helps them get a fuller understanding of you.
- Scour the world for information on your condition: Talk to everyone you know (perhaps someone plays golf with an expert!) and use the Internet to find support groups and experts, wherever they are. Don't be afraid to "cold call" experts who might be helpful.
- If you go to pain clinics, find doctors who are not only excellent scientists but who are also compassionate and who *take you seriously.* They should have a *belief* that you will get

better. Don't accept any less from your caregivers.

- Make as many appointments with different experts as you think you might need. Often these appointments take months to get, so it is better to have them and then cancel them later if you do not need them.
- Research every pain medication they want to put you on. Ask about side effects.
- Practice whatever form of meditation you are comfortable with, including slow, meditative walking. (See Chapter 14, "Meditation.")
- Practice daily one or more of: yoga, tai chi and qigong, all of which involve deep, cleansing breathing, and all of which have been useful for pain management.
- There are many forms of massage and body-work that may be helpful, including Trager® movement education, craniosacral therapy, tui na and qigong energy work, as well as Ayurvedic massage.
- Develop and maintain a healthy lifestyle by eating healthfully, controlling your weight, exercising regularly and managing stress. You can ask your doctor for referrals to a nutritionist, exercise program and stress-reduction program.
- Try to get in touch with your spirituality: Often, finding a belief in a higher power or some universal source of healing can help make the

unbearable more bearable. Take time to explore issues of purpose and meaning in your life.

- Try to understand, through psychotherapy, paying attention to your dreams or by using your journal, any deeper message that the pain might have about your life, your relationship to your body or your relationships to those who are close to you. This might be a message that you have ignored or overlooked in the past.

3

INTEGRATIVE MEDICINE FOR CHRONIC PAIN: THE BEST TOOLS FROM CONVENTIONAL AND ALTERNATIVE MEDICINE

Here is a summary of both conventional and alternative treatments for chronic pain. Most will be explained more fully later in the book. Do not use any of these treatments on your own. Always consult with your doctor first. You can use this list as a tool to begin exploring options with your doctor.

Conventional Tools for Pain Control

Conventional tools for pain control include:

- *Non-steroidal anti-inflammatories* (NSAIDs), including aspirin, ibuprofen, indomethacin, naproxen. The side effects can include high blood pressure, intestinal bleeding, and liver and kidney damage.

- *Analgesics*, including the anti-inflammatories mentioned above, plus acetaminophen; and *narcotics*, such as morphine, which are by prescription only. Side effects of narcotics include drowsiness, confusion and constipation.

- *Neuropathic pain medications*, which target pain that seems to have no obvious cause, or that remains after the original injury has healed. Neuropathic pain is thought to come from the central nervous system.

- *Transcutaneous nerve stimulation (TENS)* uses a small, battery-powered stimulator to apply a gentle, painless electrical current to a certain area of the skin. The electrical current may block pain signals or cause the body to release endorphins (one of the body's natural painkillers). This technique must be done by a professional. TENS may help some people and some types of pain more than others.

- *Physical therapy* for help with posture, movement and exercise; and *occupational therapy* to help you learn ways to do work and activities more easily.

- *Heat and/or cold therapy*, under the advice of a health-care professional.

Complementary Methods of Pain Management

Complementary and alternative approaches to pain management include:

- *Regular exercise* is an important part of pain management, but you should consult with your doctor to make sure that the exercise is appropriate for your pain and your physical condition. Exercise releases endorphins (natural painkillers), strengthens muscles and bones, keeps joints more flexible, reduces stress, increases energy, improves sleep and helps with weight control. Choose activities you enjoy, start slowly and try to build up to thirty minutes of moderate exercise on most, and preferably all, days of the week.
- *Traditional Chinese Medicine (TCM)* includes several methods that studies have found effective in pain reduction. These include:
  — *Acupuncture* (which uses thin needles) and *acupressure* (manual pressure) to stimulate some of the more than 400 "acupoints" on

the body's surface. Stimulation of certain points in particular has been associated with pain reduction.

— *Traditional Chinese herbs.* The use of herbs comes from three thousand years of observation and practice. There are more than twelve thousand known plants in China that can be used as medicine, but practitioners generally use about three hundred. Always consult with your doctor and a qualified TCM practitioner before using any herbs.

— *Movement therapies.* These include qigong exercises and tai chi. These slow, meditative movements are thought to increase the flow of Qi (life force, pronounced "chi") in the body, improve energy and balance, and provide a feeling of general well-being. They teach you to associate movement with relaxation and health.

• *Bioelectric magnetic therapies* involve the use of magnets to treat pain. These therapies are primarily complementary and may be helpful for symptom management. *Magnets should be avoided if you have implanted devices such as pacemakers or artificial heart valves.*

• *Dietary changes.* For some people, avoiding

nightshade vegetables such as tomatoes, potatoes, bell peppers and eggplant, as well as dairy and wheat, has been helpful.

- *Pain-reducing herbs and supplements* include boswellia, bupleurum, celery seed, devil's claw, ginger, goldenrod, guaiac, licorice, sarsaparilla, turmeric, omega-3 fish oils, and yucca for osteoarthritis and other inflammatory conditions. Yuan Hu-So, certain types of willow bark, SAM-e (pronounced "Sammy") and capsaicin (red pepper) are used topically. B vitamins, calcium/magnesium and glucosamine sulfate are other examples of herbs and supplements that may be useful for certain painful conditions. (See Chapter 6 for details about diet and pain.) **Before using supplements, vitamins or dietary changes to treat pain, you should first consult your physicians to make sure they are safe for you.**

- *Manipulative therapies*, including most kinds of massage (especially trigger point, Shiatsu and deep tissue), chiropractic, osteopathic manipulation and craniosacral therapy.

- *Mind/body and bodywork therapies*, including the Alexander Technique, Feldenkreis, meditation, hypnosis, guided imagery, biofeedback, behavioral therapy and Trager® movement education, which uses gentle, rhythmic movements to facilitate the release of stress patterns, either on the mental, emotional or physical levels.

Osteoarthritis

Brian Berman, M.D., director of integrative medicine at the University of Maryland, describes a patient who, like Barbara in Chapter 2, took managing her pain into her own hands, combining CAM and conventional care.

Angela (not her real name), a financial analyst in her mid-forties, had osteoarthritis in her neck that was causing chronic, unrelenting pain so severe that she could barely turn her head. She had tried drugs as well as physical therapy, with little success. Examination revealed that a compressed disk in her neck was inflamed and pressing on a nerve. Other doctors had advised her that surgery was the solution, but she was reluctant to undergo an operation.

"I have found that acupuncture of the ear is often helpful for musculoskeletal problems," says Dr. Berman. (In Chinese medicine, every part of the body is represented by a point on the ear.) "I decided to begin with ear acupuncture every week to reduce the inflammation of the disk, followed by acupuncture along the 'meridians' (energy pathways) in the body that relate to the area that was inflamed." Over the next couple of months, Angela reported that her pain was reduced to the point that she felt she did not need surgery. Dr. Berman stretched out her sessions to every other week. "As we worked together, Angela and I got to know each other a little better," says Dr. Berman. "She began to talk about the 'pressure cooker' atmosphere of the world of finance, as well as family issues that were causing stress in her life. I suggested that she try meditation and relaxation exercises." Angela agreed to work with a staff member in the pain clinic to learn some techniques that she could use on her own at home. "Often, meditation and relaxation exercises help reduce some of our perceptions of pain, which, as we know, is always *subjective* in nature," says Dr. Berman. "We have found that meditation helps to modulate pain signals sent to the brain by sending other signals back to the site of the pain that, in effect, 'turn down the volume.'"

From Victim of Pain to Being in Control

Within a few months, Angela was able to manage her pain so that it no longer interfered with her life. When she had flare-ups, Dr. Berman sent her for physical therapy for exercises in mobility and strengthening that she could do at home. She learned other ways to help herself as well: improving her diet, for example, by reducing caffeine and sodas, white flour and sugar, and adding more soy, fish and complex carbohydrates. (See Chapter 6 for recent research on diet and pain.) She also began taking supplements such as calcium/magnesium and glucosamine/chondroitin sulfate, both of which have been found to reduce the symptoms of osteoarthritis.

Nine years later, Angela has still not had surgery and feels no need to do so. Her pain occurs sporadically, because the osteoarthritis is still present, but she has learned how to manage and reduce the discomfort through a program that combines acupuncture, meditation, dietary changes and exercises. She is now less a victim and more in control of the pain. *She has begun to own her health.*

An Integrative Approach to Osteoarthritis

Arthritis pain is caused by degeneration of the joints, leading to pain and inflammation. Anything you can do to strengthen the joints and reduce the inflammation will help. Here are some recommended methods from integrative medicine:

- **Movement.**
  — Physical therapy for mobility and strengthening
  — Gentle yoga
  — Traditional Chinese exercises: tai chi, qigong
- **Massage with herbal oils.** You can massage the following oils (diluted with olive oil) into unbroken skin to relieve arthritis pain. *Note that these oils are never to be taken internally.*
  — Olive oil (plain or combined with other oils)
  — Arnica oil
  — Capsaizin oil (made from red pepper)
  — Lobelia seed oil
- **Alternating hot and cold packs/soaks.** Alternate temperatures, using heat for two to three minutes and then cold for thirty seconds to one minute on painful areas.
- **Meditation for relaxation.**
- **Pulsed electromagnetic fields (EMFs).** Vary in terms of frequency (measured in hertz or oscillations per second) and strength (measured in gauss or tesla). Preliminary studies have examined the effects of both high-strength, high-frequency stimulation, and low-strength, low-frequency stimulation on

pain. Both were found to be effective in reducing the pain of osteoarthritis.

- **Fasting or elimination diets.** Fasting has been shown to influence the pain of rheumatoid arthritis. Several studies also have shown that humans with rheumatoid arthritis have temporary improvement in their joint inflammation when they fast for seven to ten days. Fasting is not a practical long-term therapy and *unsupervised fasting is dangerous.* Yet these observations lend additional support to the idea that diet affects joint inflammation and should also be considered in the treatment of osteoarthritis. (See Chapter 6 on diet and pain for more details.)

- **Energy and movement therapies.**
  - Acupuncture
  - Massage, including muscular therapy, shiatsu, trigger point, craniosacral therapy
  - The Alexander Technique

- **Supplements.** (Consult with your doctor for correct dosage and type.)
  - Bromelain with rutin and trypsin (Phlogenzym)
  - Glucosamine sulfate (Watch your blood sugar because this might increase it.)
  - Grape seed
  - MSM
  - Omega-3 fish oils

- — Pine bark
- — Quercetin (found in onion skins and many plants)
- — SAM-e
- — Vitamin C
- **Herbs.**
  - — Boswellia
  - — Bupleurum
  - — Celery seed
  - — Devil's claw
  - — Garlic
  - — Ginger
  - — Goldenrod
  - — Guaiac
  - — Oregano
  - — Red pepper
  - — Rosemary
  - — Sarsaparilla
  - — Stinging nettle
  - — Teasel
  - — Turmeric
  - — Willow
  - — Yucca

- **Foods to eat.**
  - Broccoli
  - Complex carbohydrates
  - Green tea (antioxidant)
  - Lots of fresh, colorful vegetables. The pigments of richly colored vegetables are anti-inflammatory. Botanist James A. Duke's "arthritis soup" includes cabbage, string beans, celery, stinging nettle leaves, carrots, asparagus, dandelion root, spinach, eggplant, chicory, garlic, turmeric, licorice, evening primrose seeds, ground red pepper, white mustard, flaxseed, sarsaparilla, fenugreek, lemon juice.[4] If you are not a vegetarian, Dale Bellisfield, R.N., A.H.G., recommends adding bone and gristle to soups.
  - Nontoxic fish such as sardines and herring, as well as *wild caught* salmon and fish or shellfish that are relatively low in mercury: scallops, shrimp, flounder and haddock.
  - Pineapple
  - Soy (with caution. See "The Latest Word on Soy" in Chapter 6.)
- **Foods to avoid.**
  - White flour, white rice, white potatoes, white sugar

— Soda
— Trans fats
— For some people, wheat, dairy, and "night-shades" such as tomato, potato, bell pepper and eggplant make arthritis worse.

4

THE BIOPSYCHOSOCIAL APPROACH: TREATING MORE THAN PAIN

"Biopsychosocial" is a long word, but it simply means that doctors must never forget that those aching bones or muscles are attached to a person with a life history, certain ways of coping, personal values, a family, a job, relationships and financial pressures. First described in 1984 by British surgeon Gordon Waddell, this method treats the physical symptoms of pain while also taking into account patients' beliefs, psychological stresses and attitudes toward their bodies.

This approach has been part of the conventional training of doctors for many years, but with the advent of managed care, shortened office visits and the pressures of seeing too many patients in too short a period of time, many doctors are unable to use the biopsychosocial approach with their patients. Getting to know the patient on all of these levels simply takes up too much time.

The movement toward integrative medicine—combining alternative/complementary and conventional treatments—is beginning to change the way that medicine is delivered in this country. Integrative physicians are finding the time to look at issues of mind and spirit—as well as body—with their patients, and the result, in the long run, is healthier patients and less pressure on an already overstretched health care system. When patients are helped to understand the relationship between their minds, spirits and health, and to take more responsibility for reducing stress and other life pressures, their health improves, so they may need to see the doctor less often.

TIP

Here is a list of questions that your doctor should ask you about your pain. Try to answer them now to get a better idea of your condition.

1. What is your diagnosis? Have all appropriate conventional treatments been considered?
2. What is your diet and level of nutrition, including supplements? How does this relate to your health problem? (For example, is your weight contributing to your lower back pain?)
3. What is your level of exercise? How can you engage in regular, appropriate exercise for the condition? (This is especially important when dealing with pain.)
4. How do you handle stress, either from family, job or other relationships? What emotional problems are you facing right now? What are your coping mechanisms? How can you improve your response to stress?
5. What is your spiritual belief system? Do you have an awareness of your purpose or meaning in life? Is there a balance among work, leisure, loving relationships, and appreciation of art, creativity or nature?

Here is a story to illustrate how the biopsychosocial integrative approach works: My patient was in her mid-fifties and suffering from chronic back pain that was the result of osteoporosis and several small spinal fractures from a car accident. She was in near-constant pain and could not travel, stand or sit without significant discomfort. After consulting with many conventional and alternative specialists, she eventually decided to undergo surgery. According to the surgeons who reviewed her postoperative x-rays, the surgery to repair the fractures was a complete success.

However, six months after the surgery, she still had enough pain that it was interfering with her quality of life. After getting to know her, I discovered that she had been an artist and that painting had always been a way for her to express her essence as a person. But in the last year, she had moved to a new house and had not had the energy to set up her painting studio. As a result, she was not feeling "whole," because an important part of her "self" was still not being expressed. Interestingly, the root of the word "healing" means "to make whole."

As we talked, it became clear to both of us that she needed to paint again. She set up her studio and threw herself wholeheartedly into her art once more. Within a very short time, her pain had diminished to the extent that it no longer interfered with her daily activities. By taking control of "owning" her life, she has transformed herself and found wholeness and healing.

You might have a different way to feel whole—some people find wholeness in religion or spirituality;

others in the middle of a forest or out on a sailboat; still others through listening to or playing music. But whatever it is, if you look inside yourself, perhaps with the help of your doctor or health care professional, you may well find your own personal key to healing and wholeness. What important part of your life is being denied to you because of your pain? How can you reincorporate into your life what is most important to you?

Part of this process is to look for a healing relationship with a doctor who practices integrative medicine. Through such a relationship, a doctor can understand your life and personality and treat you as a whole person, rather than just a collection of symptoms. This is particularly useful when no reason for the symptoms seems clear from the Western perspective. Is your doctor aware of your personal values and the important parts of your life that are affected by the pain? If not, try to communicate this to your doctor, either during an appointment or by writing a note or e-mail. The act of writing down some of these feelings may also help you to clarify what is going on in your life as a result of the pain.

Abdominal Pain

Erica had stomachaches growing up, but nothing like what she felt while she was trying to get pregnant with her first child. "I went to the hospital, doubled over in agony and screaming in pain," she recalls. "I had lost twenty-five pounds in one month, and the pain in my stomach had been building steadily until I could no longer tolerate it." Tests found that she had a fever and an elevated white blood count; doctors initially assumed she had appendicitis. One doctor told her the pain was "all in your mind." A sigmoidoscopy (examination of only the lower part of the large bowel) revealed nothing.

The pain finally subsided on its own, and Erica became pregnant almost immediately. "During those nine months, I felt great," she says. "I assumed that the pregnancy had somehow put whatever this disease was into a kind of remission." But four days after giving birth, she was back in the hospital again. "The pain was as bad as ever," she remembers. "Only this time I began bleeding profusely every time I had a bowel movement. The blood just came pouring out of me."

She found a new doctor. "He was wonderful," she says. "Very different. He would hop onto the table, look me in the eye and want to know about my life, about my new baby, was I happy? None of the other doctors had ever looked me in the eye before, and no one had been interested in my life."

The new doctor did something more: He decided to do a complete colonoscopy—examining the entire large bowel—that finally solved the mystery. He diagnosed Crohn's disease, a chronic digestive disorder that falls into the category of "inflammatory bowel disease" (IBD).

It is thought that Crohn's disease is caused by the body's immune system wrongly reacting to the lining of the digestive system as if it were "foreign" tissue and therefore dangerous. White blood cells rush to attack the "invader," creating holes or ulcerations in the lining of the intestine, giving it a "cobblestone" appearance. The holes cause pain and bleeding and, eventually, scar tissue, which can cause a severe, sometimes fatal obstruction of the bowel.

"I learned that Crohn's disease plays hide and seek," says Erica. "It can skip part of the intestine, which is why the first doctor never saw it. He didn't look far enough inside my intestine." The new doctor prescribed medication that helped alleviate the pain and symptoms somewhat, but did not eliminate them. "I felt a profound sense of relief that I wasn't crazy, that I finally understood what was happening in my body," says Erica. "I almost didn't care that I still had some symptoms."

Crohn's disease can lie dormant for months or years, followed by intense periods of pain and symptoms that can last an equal amount of time. Over the next several years, Erica had several debilitating bouts with the disease, requiring emergency visits to the hospital, surgery and being immobilized by pain for months at a time.

Moving into Health

Desperate to help their daughter, Erica's parents, who live in Florida, turned to the Internet, where they found the Web site of the Crohn's and Colitis Foundation of America (*www.ccfa.org*) and learned about the work of Alvin Zfass, M.D., a specialist and professor at Medical College of Virginia. "It took almost two months to get an appointment with him," says Erica. "But it was worth the wait. He saved my life in a lot of different ways."

Dr. Zfass admitted Erica to the hospital to wean her off of the steroids that had been prescribed for her but that were causing weight gain as well as debilitating muscle pain. After a couple of weeks, Erica went home and, with supervision, slowly cut down her use of steroids. "Dr. Zfass used some of the

A SECOND BRAIN IN THE GUT?
EVIDENCE SAYS YES

Ever wonder why you get butterflies in your stomach when you are nervous? In addition to the brain and central nervous system we all know about, there is evidence that a second complex "brain" and nervous system also exist in the human gut. The gut brain, called the "enteric nervous system," has been described by Michael Gershon, M.D., professor of anatomy and cell biology at Columbia Presbyterian Medical Center in New York. In a 1996 interview with *The New York Times*, Gershon explained that nearly every substance that helps run and control the brain has turned up in the gut. These include serotonin, dopamine, glutamate, norepinephrine and nitric oxide, as well as two dozen small brain proteins, called neuropeptides, and major cells of the immune system. This explains why so many emotional states affect the bowel and stomach.[5]

Dr. Gershon is considered one of the founders of a new field of medicine called "neurogastroenterology." (More information is available from the International Foundation for Functional Gastrointestinal Disorders at *www.iffgd.org*.)

newer medicines to treat the symptoms—diarrhea, ulcers and pain. Slowly, my intestines and joints healed, and after about a year, I was off the steroids completely and had begun to lose the excess weight," says Erica.

But a resurgence of severe symptoms in 2001 propelled Erica into an exploration of alternative medicine. Still coping with almost daily pain and diarrhea, Erica decided to expand her options. "I figured I had nothing to lose," she says. "Western medicine was offering me its best, but I felt I needed some additional tools." Since the beginning of her illness nearly twelve years before, Erica, like Barbara in Chapter 2, had also been doing some soul-searching on her own to try to discover the meaning of what was happening to her.

"I had read the book, *Man's Search for Meaning*, by the late psychiatrist Viktor Frankl," she says. "It changed my life. He used his experiences in Auschwitz to find meaning in the midst of suffering. I was trying to do the same thing. Why should a twenty-six-year-old girl be suffering like this? I realized that if I waited for someone to give me an answer, I'd still be waiting. I had to make sense of my suffering, and this book helped me do that." In addition to her inner explorations, Erica also started using her treadmill regularly again. "I am stubborn, and didn't want to give up exercising," she says. "I was not going to let this disease beat me."

Learning the Language of the Body

Then Erica heard about a class at a local health center called "The Nervous Stomach." "I knew that it was primarily for people with irritable bowel syndrome, which is less serious than IBD and Crohn's, so I was initially skeptical." But after consulting with the teacher, Sarena Morello, M.S., Erica decided to give the class a try.

The class included the use of biofeedback. Biofeedback training uses instruments that measure body "language," including muscle tension and finger temperature. The instruments transmit this information to us, either on a screen or with sounds. "Research and clinical practice with biofeedback has shown that we can consciously use this information to self-regulate many of the functions of the autonomic nervous system, which includes the 'automatic' functions of your body, such as heart rate, blood pressure or finger temperature," says Morello, a licensed mental health counselor and biofeedback expert who developed the program.

TIP

For details about biofeedback, autogenic training, hypnotherapy and other mind/body methods of treating pain, see Chapter 5.

"Instead of the Pain Happening to Me, I Can Make Something Happen to the Pain."

Erica knew that Crohn's disease was not likely to be cured by biofeedback alone. "But I told Sarena that I wanted another tool to use when I was in pain, and she thought it might be helpful," says Erica. "The biofeedback training, combined with the breathing, positive imagery and visualization, helped me to control my fear during pain episodes. When I am in pain, my hands and feet are freezing. Using the program, I can usually raise the temperature of my extremities by several degrees. This increased blood flow also goes back to my GI tract and seems to calm down the intestinal area. Last week, I had pain that I managed to reduce from a level of ten, the highest on my personal scale, to a level three or four. It seems to work every time."

Now, says Erica, she has more of a feeling of control over her illness. "Instead of the pain happening to me, I can make something happen to the pain," she says. "I can control my fear and separate this pain from the years of horrible pain experiences in my past. I can stay calm, which relaxes my intestines and my whole body."

Erica describes herself as her own advocate for health: "I treat doctors as people who work for me." Using a combination of conventional and alternative methods, Erica continues to make progress. In February 2005, Erica gave birth to her fourth child, at the age of forty. "My pregnancy was problem-free," she says. "Since then I have been fine. I meditate every day and try to keep stress to a minimum. I have so much joy with this new baby and that joy colors everything. In my mind, my Crohn's is gone, and I just keep moving forward positively. I drink two or three quarts of green tea daily, but no other medications, and no huge supplemental regime. For now . . . I truly feel the place I am in mentally, emotionally, spiritually, buoyed by the pregnancy, allowing me a true and full remission, is just keeping me in a very healthy place!"

TIP

When you have to go to the hospital, bring headphones, a portable CD player, and your own library of relaxation/meditation tapes with instructions on calming breathing techniques. Listen to these instead of that TV set hanging from the ceiling!

An Integrative Approach to Gastrointestinal Pain

Combining conventional and alternative methods for irritable bowel syndrome, inflammatory bowel disease (IBD) and Crohn's disease is possible if you work closely with your conventional doctor to evaluate the effects of:

- Medication
- Steroids (short-term)
- Biofeedback training
- Hypnotherapy

in conjunction with alternative treatments:
- Deep, yogic breathing and relaxation techniques
- Visualization
- Meditation
- Supplements that helped Erica with the pain of Crohn's disease: lecithin, aloe vera, acidophilus, bifidus, vitamin C (in liquid form), Greens+ (in a smoothie drink), DHA and a multivitamin with energy boosters

Herbs and Dietary Suggestions for Inflammatory Bowel Disease

Botanist James A. Duke, Ph.D., author of *The Green Pharmacy*, has the following recommendations for the treatment of IBD. Consult with your doctor before trying any of these.

- **Explore food sensitivities** to milk and dairy

products, and gluten and soy (try substituting rice cakes for bread and rice noodles for pasta).

- **Onion skins** have quercetin, the top compound with anti-IBD effects. Dr. Duke suggests putting the whole onion, skin and all, into soups and stews while they're cooking. "Just remove the parchmentlike skin at the last moment before serving."[6]

- **Psyllium** is a seed from the fleawort plant that expands when moist. Psyllium's ability to absorb fluids also makes it useful for treating diarrhea, a common IBD symptom. In addition, as it travels through the digestive tract, the mucilage in psyllium exerts a soothing effect, which may help relieve the cramping of IBD. If you use psyllium, make sure that you drink plenty of fluids and watch for allergic reactions.[7]

- **Tea**, including plain tea, as well as herb teas made with bayberry, bugleweed, bilberry, black walnut, English walnut, carob and raspberry, have astringent, tannin properties that are beneficial for relieving gastrointestinal distress.

- **Steroids** (short-term)

- **Valerian** (an herb) relieves spasms in smooth muscles such as the intestine and helps relieve stress, a contributor to IBD.

- **Massage** with a variety of diluted essential oils for relaxation (for external use only).
- **Assorted herbs, taken as tea or extract.** Chamomile, peppermint and wild yam can help relieve muscle spasms, including those of the intestine.[8]

More Problems of the Digestive Tract

The following herbs and dietary suggestions are from Dale Bellisfield, R.N., A.H.G. Check with your doctor and a certified herbalist for correct dosage and whether the herb or supplement is appropriate for you.

- **General abdominal pain.** Try to keep your bowels regular and avoid eating trans fats. The following herbs may help: black cohosh, corydalis, Chinese white peony, cramp bark, cyperus, dang gui, Jamaica dogwood, ligusticum, PA-free petasites (butterbur), Roman chamomile. You may also want to try the following supplements: magnesium, omega-3, B complex, calcium, bromelain, quercetin, probiotics.
- **Inflammatory Bowel Disease.** Slippery elm, licorice, turmeric, sarsaparilla, wild yam, Roman chamomile, marshmallow, meadowsweet, prickly

ash, yarrow (mucous colitis), calendula, kudzu root, cyperus, una de gato, myrrh.

- **Autoimmune digestive disorders.** Maitake, reishi, ashwugandha, cordyceps, licorice.
- **H. pylori.** Blueberry, cranberry, goldenseal, oregano, rosemary, sage.
- **Constipation.** Fenugreek seed, triphala, flaxseed, psyllium seeds, slippery elm.
- **Diarrhea.** Astringents: Oregon grape (berberines), coptis, yellow root, goldenseal.
- **Ulcerative colitis.** Boswellia.
- **Gastritis and ulcers.** Raw potato juice with raw cabbage juice/chickweed juice.
- **Gastroesophageal reflux disease (GERD).** Avoid mints, carbonated drinks, alcohol, chocolate, acidic food, cigarettes.

Foods to Improve Digestion and Reduce Pain

- **Probiotic foods.** These are nonpasteurized fermented foods that support digestive functioning and reduce abdominal pain by providing beneficial digestive bacteria.
  — Kimchee
  — Miso
  — Natto

- — Plain kefir
- — Sauerkraut
- — Tempeh
- — Yogurt
- **Prebiotic Foods.** These support digestive functioning and increase healing.
  - — Banana
  - — Black beans
  - — Jerusalem artichokes
- **Soothing foods.** These foods help to heal painful ulcerations of mucus membranes from the mouth through the whole digestive tract.
  - — Cinnamon
  - — Flaxseed
  - — Kudzu root
  - — Okra
- **Fragrant spices.** These are anti-inflammatory, antioxidant, antiviral and antibacterial and relieve gas, nausea, belching and rumbling.
  - — Anise
  - — Basil
  - — Caraway
  - — Cardamom
  - — Cilantro
  - — Cinnamon
  - — Cloves
  - — Coriander

— Dill
— Fennel
— Lavender
— Rosemary
— Sage
— Thyme
- **Other digestive aids.**
  — Kiwi
  — Mango
  — Papaya
  — Pineapple

Foods That May Contribute to Abdominal Pain

Avoid the following: gluten grains, dairy, coffee, trans fats, soy, pork, lamb, junk foods, high-fat foods and any suspected allergens.

5

BIOFEEDBACK AND HYPNOTHERAPY FOR PAIN

Think of putting a piece of freshly cut lemon into your mouth. Do you begin to salivate? There is obviously no lemon in your mouth, but your body has changed its chemistry to act is if there were. Your mind has a powerful ability to affect your body, according to Gary L. Goldberg, Ph.D., a clinical psychologist who specializes in health psychology. For the past thirty years, Dr. Goldberg has successfully used a number of mind/body techniques, including biofeedback and hypnotherapy, to help patients overcome pain as well as many other health problems. He is currently practicing at the Siegler Center for Integrative Medicine at St. Barnabas Hospital in New Jersey.

"Research shows that positive thoughts create positive chemistry inside the body, and negative thoughts create negative chemistry," says Dr. Goldberg. "When we have angry thoughts or are upset, our bodies produce stress hormones such as adrenalin and cortisol, which cause scores of chemical reactions that prepare us for 'fight or flight.' This response is 'hardwired' into our bodies, because when we were living in caves, it was adaptive. It helped people survive when they were chased by saber-toothed tigers, for example."

But in modern life, the "fight or flight" response can be destructive to our health, says Dr. Goldberg. "Your metabolism stops; your heart beats faster; your breathing quickens; your pupils dilate; your blood pressure goes up; your muscles tighten—all preparing you to fight or run. If you are in pain, this 'fight or flight' response will make your pain worse."

The opposite reaction to the "fight or flight" response is the "relaxation response," a term coined by Herbert Benson, M.D., Harvard Medical School, to describe a state that can be achieved through meditation. "The goal of all of my work with mind/body techniques is to help my patients learn to create a relaxation response," says Dr. Goldberg.

"Unlike the 'fight or flight' response, the 'relaxation response' is not hardwired into our bodies. So it has to be learned." Dr. Goldberg describes the relaxation response state as one that increases "alpha" brain waves, which appear as slow, regular and symmetrically curved. (When you are feeling stress or anger, other, less healthful waves predominate).

Dr. Goldberg teaches his patients to activate the relaxation response in order to diminish their pain through such methods as biofeedback, autogenic training, guided imagery, hypnotherapy and diaphragmatic breathing. "I match the method I use to the person," says Dr. Goldberg. "If someone is more comfortable with computers and machines, I use biofeedback. For someone who likes to solve problems alone, autogenic training with diaphragmatic breathing or meditation may be more appropriate. And for people who like to connect with others, I use guided imagery or hypnotherapy. But no matter what the method, the goal is the same: to create a state of deep relaxation and peace, with the brain in an 'alpha' state and the body comfortable and experiencing less pain."

Biofeedback

Biofeedback does not "do" anything to you. It is what you do inside your own mind and body when you receive information from the biofeedback instruments that makes the difference. During a typical session, a sensor will be placed on your finger and connected to a computer, which can then measure your heart rate, the temperature of your skin and your blood pressure. "These are bodily responses that are normally not in our conscious control, because they are regulated by the autonomic nervous system," says Dr. Goldberg. "But we have found that with training, patients can voluntarily self-regulate the operations of the autonomic nervous system: cardiovascular (heart), gastrointestinal (gut), immune, respiratory (breathing) and circulatory (blood flow)."

You might, for example, see an image on the computer screen that shows a sun rising or setting, depending on the level of your blood pressure; a clown juggling balls faster or slower, depending on how fast your heart is beating; changes on a thermometer to indicate whether increased blood flow to your hands is making them warmer; or jagged or straight brain wave lines depending on your state of mind. "Through biofeedback, patients can learn to respond to these computer images and then change them by actually changing the functioning of their bodies, even if they can't describe exactly how they made these changes," says Dr. Goldberg.

Autogenic Training

Two German psychologists, Wolfgang Luthe and Johannes H. Schultz, developed autogenic training in 1932. Autogenic training—like some forms of meditation—helps you develop an internal awareness, allowing you to observe your thoughts and feelings without judging them or getting caught up in them. The technique involves the repetition of phrases in order to relax muscles, visceral organs and body tissue. "The basis of autogenic training is that if you think something is happening, your brain can make it happen," says Dr. Goldberg. "The method trains people to use their own inner resources to help themselves."

In a typical session, Dr. Goldberg helps patients to relax through special breathing techniques (see "Diaphragmatic Breathing" in this chapter), and then to imagine the arms and legs feeling warm and very heavy. "When you imagine this while in a relaxed state, your blood vessels will expand, bringing more blood and oxygen to your muscles, which then cause the muscles to release any spasm that is causing pain," says Dr. Goldberg. "When muscles are deprived of oxygen, they go into spasm and cause pain. Another benefit of this technique is that it increases the efficiency of insulin to carry sugars out of the bloodstream and into the body tissues that use it to function properly."[9]

Diaphragmatic Breathing

"If you have ever watched a newborn breathe, you know what diaphragmatic breathing is," says Dr. Goldberg. "Only their stomachs go up and down because they are breathing from the deepest part of the abdomen. This is the healthiest way to breathe." But most of us learn very early to abandon this form of breathing for the shallower "thoracic" or chest breathing. "When we are stressed, we take very shallow breaths from our chest, and this brings less oxygen into our bodies, which can cause muscle tightness, pain and even anxiety," says Dr. Goldberg.

During all mind/body work, Dr. Goldberg encourages his patients to engage in diaphragmatic breathing to bring more oxygen into the body and induce relaxation, in preparation for autogenic training, guided imagery, hypnotherapy or meditation. But even if you are not in a mind/body training session, you can use diaphragmatic breathing on your own whenever you feel stressed, anxious or in pain.

RELAXATION PHRASES YOU CAN USE

In his autogenic training sessions, Dr. Gary Goldberg teaches patients to use the following sequence of phrases to help them relax. These can be helpful when you are in pain.

Close your eyes, breathe deeply and repeat the following phrases slowly to yourself while allowing yourself to feel the sensations:

- My left arm and hand are feeling warm.
- My right arm and hand are feeling warm.
- My left arm and hand are feeling heavy.
- My right arm and hand are feeling heavy.
- My left foot and leg are feeling warm.
- My right foot and leg are feeling warm.
- My left foot and leg are feeling heavy.
- My right foot and leg are feeling heavy.
- My arms and legs are feeling warm and heavy.
- I am feeling calm, peaceful and relaxed.

Biofeedback and Autogenic Training: What's the Evidence?

Biofeedback may benefit people with chronic pain, headaches, elevated blood pressure, asthma and many other conditions, especially in combination with relaxation methods. Research shows that both autogenic training (including relaxation, visualization and autosuggestion) and biofeedback have been found to be effective in the treatment of certain conditions, including gastrointestinal disorders and insomnia. Systematic reviews of clinical trials (including observational studies) of biofeedback in tension headaches and migraines in adults and children found that the combination of biofeedback and relaxation is more effective than either therapy used alone.[10]

In his book, *The Best Alternative Medicine: What Works? What Does Not?* Dr. Kenneth Pelletier, former director of the Complementary and Alternative Medicine Program at Stanford University Medical School, cites several additional studies showing the effectiveness of biofeedback.[11]

Guided Imagery

For people who are comfortable being guided by someone else's voice, Dr. Goldberg recommends guided imagery. "An expert in this field named Martin Rossman has said that the processes of worrying yourself sick and imagining yourself well are quite similar," says Dr. Goldberg. "Your brain doesn't know the difference between what you are imagining and what is actually happening, so it is quite possible to imagine that your pain is leaving." As an example, Dr. Goldberg describes how he helps patients—including children—use guided imagery to reduce their pain. "I ask people to imagine stuffing all of their pain into a red helium balloon and then letting go of the string. As the balloon floats up into the sky, its color grows more and more faint, from red to cool white, as the pain is carried away." Other guided images may depend on the nature of the pain the patient is feeling. "If it feels burning hot, I help them imagine the water of a cool mountain stream pouring over it; if it is cold, they might imagine lying on a beach, being warmed by the sun. But whatever you imagine, the imagery in your brain directly affects your physiology and therefore your experience of pain."

Hypnotherapy

In the same way that consciously guided images affect the physiology of your body and your pain, your subconscious mind can also change your internal chemistry, says Dr. Goldberg. "Hypnotherapy is very different from stage hypnosis," he points out. "In a typical hypnotherapy session, the therapist will use induction to create a state of deep relaxation, during which your subconscious mind is open to suggestions that can have a powerful effect on your body. Of course, this will only work if the suggestions parallel something that you already wish for, such as a reduction of your pain."

When you are in pain, Dr. Goldberg might ask your subconscious mind to accept the fact that one of your arms is numb and that it has the power to create numbness in whatever part of your body that it touches. "I leave my patients with a posthypnotic suggestion that whenever they feel pain in the future, they can touch the painful area with the numbness-inducing arm and eliminate the pain sensation," says Dr. Goldberg. "This technique will not work for everyone, depending on their reactions to hypnotherapy, but most people will experience a positive impact."

Julietta Appleton, a certified hypnotherapist, describes the hypnotic state as one that is "a natural, delicious, relaxed feeling that many people have on a daily basis. For example, when you first wake up or just before you fall asleep or when you have a powerful emotional response to a movie or TV show." When Appleton works with clients in chronic pain she uses hypnotherapy to "teach how to turn the volume and intensity down." She does this by having the client create an image of the pain and then manipulate it, shrinking it or throwing it away. She believes there are many ways that hypnotherapy can help people control pain, especially chronic pain like fibromyalgia. "I may ask people when they are in a hypnotic state to ask for advice from their 'inner healer,' because often our subconscious minds know what our bodies need before our conscious minds do," she says. "I may also do 'parts therapy' where I'll ask the client what their emotional, intellectual, physical and spiritual parts need."

One client, for example, who had been having severe back pain, reported while under hypnosis that the emotional part of her needed to say good-bye to a baby that she had miscarried. "I had never acknowledged the pregnancy or the loss," said the client. Appleton then created a hypnotic experience in line with the client's subconscious needs: "While she was under hypnosis, I used guided imagery to help her imagine herself shrinking, traveling through her bloodstream into her uterus, connecting to the spirit of her baby and letting it know that it was loved. She sobbed through the whole process, but when she came out of her hypnotized state, the back pain was gone. She has been pain free for two years."

CAUTIONS

Check with your primary care doctor before undergoing any mind/body therapy, and make sure you work only with therapists who are certified. If you have a psychiatric disorder, always check with your mental health provider before using any of the techniques described in this chapter.

6

DIET: THE RELATIONSHIP BETWEEN FOOD AND PAIN

There are many ways to use food—particularly plants—as medicine for pain. Unlike some prescription pharmaceuticals, foods and herbs generally do not have unpleasant or dangerous side effects when used appropriately. They are also easily absorbed and used by your body. "Herbs are very safe and effective for pain relief when used with the guidance and consultation of a qualified herbalist," says Dale Bellisfield, R.N., A.H.G., who combines her medical background with certification by the American Herbalists Guild in her clinical practice at the Siegler Center for Integrative Medicine in New Jersey. Bellisfield consults with doctors and patients to determine the best foods and herbal medicines for a variety of health problems, including chronic pain. "I draw from a number of medical traditions—European herbal medicine, Traditional Chinese Medicine and Native American healing practices—to create a personalized combination of herbs, supplements, diet and lifestyle changes for each patient's condition," says Bellisfield.

Treating Pain with Diet

Dale Bellisfield's dietary and herb suggestions for specific pain conditions are included in the chapters on those conditions. Below is a summary of the properties of particular herbs and foods that she recommends for the treatment of pain.

CAUTIONS

Do not use herbs at the same time as prescription medicines; wait at least three hours. Always consult with your doctor and herbalist before taking herbs to determine the correct plant, dose and frequency, and to check for allergies. This is especially important if you are pregnant, nursing, taking prescription medicines or have any chronic conditions. Avoid smoking.

Foods to Avoid If You Are in Pain

- *Trans fats* interfere with the metabolism of essential fatty acids (such as omega-3s) that reduce inflammation and pain. They also lower HDL ("good" cholesterol) and raise LDL ("bad" cholesterol).
- *Junk foods and highly processed foods* increase inflammation and deplete nutrients.
- *Coffee* constricts blood vessels, depletes calcium and magnesium, interrupts REM sleep and stresses the adrenal glands, all of which can contribute to pain.
- *Sugar* raises adrenaline, activates inflammatory processes, suppresses immune function and thickens blood.
- *Soda drinks and sweetened juices* contain high fructose corn syrup, which interferes with collagen (essential for connective tissue) and depletes calcium. Artificial sweeteners also may increase gastrointestinal pain.

Foods to Limit If You Are in Pain

- Animal foods.
- White flour foods, white sugar, white potatoes.

- Toxic fish (Shark, swordfish, tuna, halibut, orange roughy, striped bass and snapper are examples of fish that contain high levels of mercury).
- Nightshades (for some people): tomatoes, potatoes, bell peppers, eggplant.

Foods to Eat More Of

All fragrant spices

Asparagus

Avocados

Cayenne

Chamomile

Cinnamon

Cranberries/blueberries

Fresh nuts and seeds

Fresh-ground flax seeds

Garlic

Ginger

Green tea

Horseradish

Kiwi

Mango

Olive oil

Onions

Papayas

Pineapple

Richly colored fruits and vegetables

Sardines

Seaweeds

Turmeric

Wild meats

Wild salmon

Herbs That Reduce Inflammation Pain

These herbs may be helpful for osteoarthritis, muscle pain, menstrual cramps and fibromyalgia:

Boswellia
Bupleurum
Celery seed
Devil's claw
Ginger
Goldenrod
Guaiac
Licorice
Sarsaparilla
Turmeric
Yucca

Antispasmodic Herbs

These herbs may relieve cramps, muscle spasm, some headaches and abdominal pain:

Black cohosh
Black haw
Butterbur (Petasites)
California poppy
Chinese white peony
Corydalis
Cramp bark
Gambir
Kava
Kudzu
Lobelia (herb and seed)
Roman chamomile
Skunk cabbage
Stephania
Valerian

Analgesics

The following are general pain-reducing herbs:

Black birch
Clematis
Mulberry
Poplar

Corydalis
Indian pipe
Jamaica dogwood
Meadowsweet

Willow
Wintergreen
Yellow sweet clover

Essential Oils That Reduce Pain

Essential oils are not for internal use. Dilute any of the following in olive oil and massage on unbroken skin:

Chamomile
Juniper
Lavender

Sweet birch
Wintergreen

Calming and Sedating Herbs

The following herbs have calming properties. Those marked with an asterisk (*) taste good as teas.

Blue vervain
California poppy
*Chamomile
*Fresh oat extract
Gambir
Hops
*Lavender

*Lemon balm
*Linden
Motherwort
Passionflower
Scullcap
Valerian
Wood betony

Antioxidant Foods

These foods help clear your body of free radicals and other toxins that can damage cells and cause joint pain and inflammation throughout the body:

- Fresh nuts and seeds
- Green tea
- Homemade soups cooked with bones and gristle (especially good for osteoarthritis)
- Olive oil
- Richly colored fruits and vegetables
- Horseradish (especially good for joint pain)

Probiotic Foods

Probiotics are nonpasteurized fermented foods that support digestive functioning and reduce abdominal pain by providing beneficial digestive bacteria:

Kimchee	Sauerkraut
Miso	Tempeh
Natto	Yogurt
Plain kefir	

Soothing Foods

These foods help to heal painful ulcerations of mucus membranes from the mouth through the whole digestive tract:

Cinnamon	Kudzu root
Flaxseed	Okra

Fragrant Spices for Intestinal Discomfort

These are anti-inflammatory, antioxidant, antiviral and antibacterial and relieve gas, nausea, belching and rumbling:

Anise	Coriander
Basil	Dill
Caraway	Fennel
Cardamom	Lavender
Cilantro	Rosemary
Cinnamon	Sage
Cloves	Thyme

For Constipation

Fenugreek seed	Slippery elm
Flaxseed	Triphala
Psyllium seeds	

Other Digestive Aids

Kiwi

Papaya

Mango

Pineapple

The Latest Word on Soy

There are now concerns that unfermented soy in large amounts may have a long-term negative impact, so use tofu and soymilk (both unfermented) in moderation, and check with your doctor if you have an estrogen-sensitive type of cancer before eating soy. You should also be aware that soy is highly allergenic and soy isoflavones may inhibit thyroid synthesis.

That being said, there are dietary benefits to soy. It lowers cholesterol, and certain types of soy, such as calcium-processed tofu, may be a good source of calcium, which may provide long-term protection from pain.

Fermented soy is the healthiest choice, as this is the type of soy used for thousands of years in Japan. Newer forms of soy and soy supplements do not yet have solid research behind them to determine health benefits and risks. You can buy fermented soy as miso, natto and tempeh.

7

ACUPUNCTURE AND TRADITIONAL CHINESE MEDICINE: RESTORING THE FLOW

One of Cheng Xiao Ming's most vivid memories early in his medical career was the day he examined a woman who had been injured in a car accident. He was working in a hospital in Hongzhou, China, after having graduated from a Western-style medical school (also in China) with a degree in orthopedic surgery. "My patient had a blockage in the flow of blood in her leg that had created a large stasis [pool of blood] the size of a tennis ball and hard as a rock," he remembers. He could not help her with Western methods of surgery.

In China, almost all hospitals have a system called "three legs walking," explains Cheng. "One leg is pure Western methods, one pure Traditional

Chinese Medicine (TCM) and one combined. Usually, the combined approach uses Western diagnostic methods and TCM treatment. But there are even differences in diagnosis: Western medicine diagnoses and treats a disease. TCM diagnoses by symptom, using more than twelve different wrist pulses, the condition of the tongue, and palpating (feeling) muscles and other tissues along meridians."

In most Chinese hospitals, Western-trained physicians practice alongside doctors of TCM, and this was the case in Cheng's hospital. "I watched as a TCM doctor gave the patient herbs and used his hands to move the stagnant blood," says Cheng. "In time, the herbs and the deep 'acupressure' of his hands completely resolved the stasis. This made a very deep impression in my mind."

After these experiences, Cheng decided to return to medical school, this time to study TCM. "I wanted to learn how to treat people without the side effects and pain of Western surgery," he says. Four years later, he graduated with a second medical degree and expertise in a system that was completely different from Western medicine. "Chinese medicine understands the body as a complete system— every organ and tissue has a relationship to every other, to the body as a whole, and also to the environment and even the universe," he says. "Western medicine understands the body only in relation to itself, which is, of course, useful in the diagnosis and treatment of trauma and acute problems, but limited in the treatment of chronic conditions."

Thanks to many years of teaching experience, Cheng is accustomed to explaining TCM philosophy and theory to the Western mind. "I ask my students, 'Who lives longer, the rabbit or the turtle?' They all answer, 'The turtle, of course,'" Cheng says. "Then I ask them, 'So does this mean we should all live like turtles?' 'Of course not!' they say. 'We'd never get anywhere.'"

At this point, his eyes twinkle. "Then I say to them, 'On the outside, we should be like a rabbit, strengthening our muscles, exercising our bodies and running when we need to. But on the inside, we should be like a turtle, breathing slowly and deeply, slowing the heart when it is at rest, creating a peaceful internal environment. Just like we have to train our bodies to be strong, we must also train our minds and internal organs to relax. When you are peaceful, you can logically and calmly resolve any problem, even if there is turmoil around you.'"

Qi: Universal Energy

According to TCM, blockages in the flow of "Qi" (pronounced chi)—universal energy—inside the body cause disease and pain. You can increase the flow of Qi through qigong and tai chi exercises—slow, graceful movements that Cheng calls "internal training" that help to slow down the mind and move Qi inside the body. By changing the inner environment of the body, both of these forms of exercise are thought to improve the actual functions of organs and tissues.

TIP

People usually learn qigong and tai chi under the guidance of a master teacher. But in most cities, classes in both techniques are also available in specialized centers, adult education programs and even in conventional health clubs.

It is the flow of Qi along pathways called "meridians" inside the body that is the focus of all Chinese medical treatments. Even though meridians are invisible, thousands of years of practice and observation have resulted in clearly mapped diagrams of their routes within the body. If you have ever had acupuncture and felt the tingling sensation along a meridian when a tiny needle is inserted into just the right spot, you would think that the meridians must indeed be as visible and tangible as your blood vessels. "The needles don't cure disease," explains Cheng. "They adjust the Qi, reinforcing it, reducing it where necessary, moving stagnant or 'stuck' energy. With the free flow of energy restored, the body can heal itself. After all, our bodies fight off viruses and bacteria every day. TCM methods increase that ability."

Other TCM methods include the use of Chinese herbs, taken internally or put directly on the skin; deep tissue massage (called tui na); and qigong massage (during which the practitioner uses the hands to transmit and move Qi energy with the patient fully clothed). Due to his dual training, Cheng believes in the combination of TCM with conventional Western medicine. He works regularly with patients who are also receiving conventional treatments for many conditions, including orthopedic problems, pain, cancer and stroke.

"In order for a person to get sick, the body must first have an energy deficiency, according to Chinese medicine," says Cheng. "If your body is strong everywhere, you won't get disease." Using osteoarthritis as an example, Cheng explains that internal deficiencies permit cold and damp to enter the body as pathogenic (disease-causing) infectors. "So we nourish the inside of the body with herbs so that it is strong enough to repel the cold and damp. Then we use acupuncture to restore the active function of the joints and limbs."

Traditional Chinese Medicine: What's the Evidence?

Traditional Chinese Medicine is a well-developed, coherent system of medicine that has been practiced in China for thousands of years. "As an extensive and established medical system, TCM is used by billions of people around the world for every condition known to humankind," writes Lixing Lao, Ph.D., L.Ac., associate professor in the Department of Complementary Medicine, University of Maryland School of Medicine.[12] Lao has surveyed the literature on TCM, noting, "Modern research on TCM is still in its infancy." Still, he identifies several studies that indicate TCM's usefulness as both primary and complementary therapy. These include research findings that TCM is useful in the treatment of addictions, back pain, muscle spasms and neck pain, eczema,

TRADITIONAL CHINESE MEDICINE: SUMMARY

Based on restoring the flow of energy or "Qi" throughout the body, Traditional Chinese Medicine was developed more than five thousand years ago. Qi flows along invisible pathways (meridians) in the body, and blockages in these pathways are thought to be the cause of disease and pain. TCM uses several methods to remove these blockages and restore the free flow of Qi:

- *Acupuncture:* the insertion of tiny needles at strategic points along the meridians. There is usually no pain. After the needles are inserted, you relax on the table for twenty to thirty minutes. The sensation is one of deep relaxation. People often sleep during this time and wake up refreshed. Some practitioners use laser light on the acupuncture points instead of needles.
- *Acupressure:* The practitioner uses hands to massage and exert pressure on acupuncture points.
- *Qigong and tai chi:* Slow, gentle movements that you can do yourself to strengthen your own Qi. In addition, some practitioners use qigong to transmit energy to their patients.
- *Chinese herbal medicine:* A highly evolved system that uses plants and herbs to treat disease and pain, precisely matching herbs to symptoms.

osteoarthritis, and to improve well-being.

Low back pain is the most common cause of activity limitations in people younger than forty-five and the second most frequent reason for visits to the doctor.[13] Significant new research, published in 2005, synthesized the data from thirty-three randomized, controlled trials of acupuncture for the treatment of low back pain. This broad survey (called a "meta-analysis") concluded that acupuncture effectively relieves low back pain, although there was no evidence to suggest that it was more effective than other "active" therapies.[14]

Another recent study demonstrating the effectiveness of acupuncture for osteoarthritis has stirred considerable interest in the medical community. Brian Berman, M.D., and his colleagues at the University of Maryland found that patients with osteoarthritis of the knee experienced significantly greater improvement in mobility and pain than a control group that was given "sham" acupuncture.[15]

As a therapy used in conjunction with conventional medicine, acupuncture has been found effective in such conditions as cancer pain, nausea and vomiting;[16] fibromyalgia;[17] ischemic heart disease;[18] migraine;[19] and stroke rehabilitation.[20] Lao also notes that the World Health Organization has listed over forty conditions for which acupuncture is listed as a primary or adjunctive therapy.

Lao's most poetic citation, however, comes not

from the modern research literature, but from *The Yellow Emperor's Classic of Medicine*, thought to be the first work on Traditional Chinese Medicine, published about 2,500 years ago

> In a peaceful calm,
> Void and emptiness,
> The authentic Qi
> Flows easily.
> Essences and spirits
> Are kept within.
> How could illness arise?

Fibromyalgia

There are questions about the causes of fibromyalgia—a chronic disorder characterized by widespread pain, tender points in specific parts of the body, and stiffness of muscles and associated connective tissue structures, which is typically accompanied by nonrestorative sleep, fatigue and depression. But there is no question about the misery of those who suffer from it. Here is the story of one patient who used integrative medicine to overcome fibromyalgia.

Dancing Again: Stress Management, Acupuncture, Nutrition, Exercise

My patient was in her early forties and had lived a fairly stressful life. When she was in her mid-twenties, she had had some low back pain that had resolved with rest and medication. However, in her late thirties, she was at home taking something off a high shelf when a heavy box fell onto the back of her neck. There was no fracture, but she had bruised her neck muscles. Her conventional doctor advised rest and anti-inflammatory medication, as well as physical therapy, but nothing seemed to relieve the pain.

Over time, the neck pain began to spread throughout her body, and she began feeling discomfort in her arms, legs and lower back. Sitting, standing and even sleeping became difficult, and she had trouble concentrating. Most distressing of all to her, she could not longer do things she and her husband used to enjoy: travel, dancing, going for long walks. She became depressed (understandably!) and this added to her woes.

Eventually, a rheumatologist diagnosed fibromyalgia, which can often be triggered by an emotional or physical stressor. By the time she came to see me, she was taking a tricyclic antidepressant medication, which was helping neither the pain nor the depression. She was also taking a sleeping medication and ibuprofen and had gained forty pounds, which made it even more difficult for her to move around.

I explained to her that in dealing with a condition like fibromyalgia, we need to focus on her whole self, not just the parts that hurt, and I asked if she was willing to try this approach. She agreed at once, so we began by examining her coping and stress-management skills. With the help of a psychologist, she learned visualization and progressive relaxation techniques, as well as ways in which she could identify and care for her emotional needs. We also began her on a moderate exercise program. (Aerobic exercise has been shown to be beneficial to fibromyalgia patients.)

The next step was to refer her for nutrition counseling for weight management and help with changing to a more healthful diet. I also referred her for ten sessions of acupuncture as well as to a massage therapist. Throughout this process, we continually discussed her spirituality and her sense of self, trying to determine ways to put more meaning back into her life and improve her relationships, especially with her husband. With her growing awareness of herself and what was important to her, she set a goal: She wanted to dance again with her husband.

After several months, she had lost the weight and had weaned herself from the acupuncture, except when the pain flared up. One day, she came into my office to tell me that the previous weekend she had felt well enough to go to a wedding with her husband and had danced with him for the first time in years. She cried during that dance, as did several family members who had known what she had been going through. In telling me the story, she cried again. She told me that she and her husband had started taking long walks together again and were planning a romantic trip together. Along with her renewed sense of self and control over her life, she is also now able to manage her pain without drugs and with a maintenance program of exercise, occasional acupuncture and massage. She has taken back her life.

An Integrative Approach to Fibromyalgia

- Consider psychotherapy with cognitive-behavioral and mind/body therapy as a way to manage stress and chronic pain more effectively.
- Hypnotherapy for fibromyalgia has proven benefits.[21] It decreases pain and improves sleep, as well as increases motivation to exercise and improve nutrition. It also reduces

anxiety and helps the bodily systems work together more harmoniously.

- Check with your doctor about medication or herbs for relaxation and to help you sleep.
- Try to meditate every day—even if only for a few minutes, to reduce stress (see Chapter 14 on meditation).
- Consider gentle massage, trigger point injections, Trager® movement education and craniosacral therapy.
- Several studies and anecdotal evidence suggest that acupuncture may be helpful. At least ten treatments are required.
- Focus on fresh fruits and vegetables, whole grains, low-fat sources of protein, nuts and seeds, and drink plenty of herbal teas, especially green tea and fresh water to flush toxins out of your body.
- Herbs and supplements: black cohosh, ashwugandha, kava, wood betony, omega-3, SAMe, pine bark, grape seed, quercetin. **Consult with your doctor first.**
- Some people benefit from medications such as tricyclic antidepressants and serotonin reuptake inhibitor antidepressants. Also consider acetaminophen and NSAIDS. **Discuss these options with your doctor. Avoid narcotics.**

- Movement. Regular aerobic exercise has been shown to help fibromyalgia patients. Also consider:
  — Yoga, especially the breathing and stretching techniques
  — Tai chi
  — The Alexander Technique
- Check to make sure you do not have prolonged exposure to toxic fumes in your home or workplace. Some research has linked chemical sensitivity to both fibromyalgia and chronic fatigue syndrome.[22] What are now being called "sick buildings" expose their occupants to toxic fumes from solvents, pesticides, combustion products and other irritants and petrochemicals. Many of these toxic fumes are made more dangerous by their lack of odor and the fact that prolonged exposure (such as at work every day) can cause permanent neurological damage.[23]

8

THE ALEXANDER TECHNIQUE: USING THE MIND TO FREE THE BODY FROM PAIN

Susan's chronic back pain was so severe that she needed large doses of medication and almost daily epidural injections in order to numb her spine just to get through her day. She had endured this pain for ten years. Susan (not her real name), a psychiatrist in her early thirties, had seen many specialists and had numerous tests, but no one could identify the cause. Finally, one of her doctors suggested that she try the Alexander Technique.

This method of using your body effortlessly was created out of necessity. At the turn of the twentieth century, a Shakespearean actor named Frederick M. Alexander had begun to lose his voice with increasing frequency whenever he stepped onstage. By watching himself closely in the mirror as he prepared to perform before an audience, he observed that he had developed a habit of tightening his head and neck muscles and contracting his head backward into his shoulders before each speech, compressing his larynx. When he recognized this pattern, he used close observation to develop a way of "nondoing": of freeing tension throughout the body—especially in the head and neck—by releasing any muscles that were not necessary in the activity. The technique became a way to promote effortless movement in all activities.

All Alexander practitioners refer to themselves as teachers and the people who come to them for help as students. The process is an educational one: "I don't 'cure' anyone," says Deborah Adams, who likes to be known as Debi. "I teach them, giving them the awareness and the tools to heal themselves. At the end of Susan's first lesson it became clear to me that she was making choices that were causing her difficulty," says Debi. "But these were choices that she was not even aware of." Debi had asked Susan to sit in a chair and simulate her movements during a psychotherapy session with one of her patients. As Susan did this, Debi placed her hands on Susan's shoulders and back, in the area where she felt the greatest muscle tension, and simply waited. "As I wait, I have the intention of allowing her body to release any holding patterns and lengthen, and eventually, it did so," says Debi. Alexander teachers are trained to use their hands to "listen" for tension and to gently guide release in their students. The goal is to restore the natural relationship of the head, neck and back, as Alexander had discovered.

Learning to Move with Effortless Ease

Watching Debi is itself a lesson in the Alexander Technique. Whether she is rising from a chair, walking across a room or reaching up to get a book from a shelf, her body seems to move as one fluid whole. There are no wasted motions. The head is poised gracefully on the neck, and the whole impression is one of effortless ease—almost as if she is floating without the pull of gravity. And this is exactly what it feels like during an Alexander lesson with her. You want to package up that floating feeling, carry it off with you and release it the next time you need to trudge up a flight of stairs. If you have the patience to stick with the lessons, you eventually learn to do just that.

As Debi worked with her, Susan began to notice that as she listened to her psychiatric patients, most of whom were in severe emotional distress, she had a habit of tightening her back, making it narrower and causing her head and neck to compress downward. For years, she had been unconsciously responding to her patients' distress by clenching her own back. Over the course of several lessons, she became aware of that habitual response, as well as the feeling of release when she let that response go. "The moment she learned to 'inhibit' her habitual tightening, I felt her back become wider and her spine actually lengthen," says Debi. "This freed her neck and head as well. In time, she was able to remember that feeling of release during the course of the day, and she could make the choice to allow it to happen." After several weekly lessons, Susan was gradually able to cut down on her pain medications. She no longer needs regular lessons and continues to be free of medication.

What Is the Alexander Technique?

The technique helps you gain awareness of how your mind influences the use of your body. The Alexander Technique is based on three main principles:

- Function is affected by use.
- The organism functions as a whole.
- The relationship of the head, neck and spine is vital to the organism's ability to function optimally.

During an Alexander lesson, you remain fully clothed. Depending on the nature of your pain, the teacher may have you simply sit on a chair or stand or move between the two positions; at some point in the lesson, you may also lie down on a table. You are encouraged to bring any of your daily activities to a lesson; musicians can, for example, bring in their instruments. During a lesson, the teacher places her hands on your body—neck, shoulders, arms, legs, back or hips—and simply waits, "listening" to find out where there is tightness or where the body is not functioning as a whole. As she does this, your attention is brought to where she has placed her hands, and you might begin to release muscles that you did not even know you were contracting. You might realize, for example, "I don't need to hunch my shoulders in order to stand up, I can release them and simply use my leg muscles." You are doing what Alexander teachers call "inhibition" or interception of a habitual response. With time, this kind of awareness carries over into everyday activities, with the result that you use your body differently, with less effort and with less pain.

Conditions most frequently treated with the Alexander Technique include chronic pain, osteoarthritis, stress and headaches. It is also common for musicians, dancers, singers and actors to use the technique to improve their performances onstage.

The Alexander Technique: What's the Evidence?

Research has found that the Alexander Technique is useful for breathing, chronic pain, daily function, Parkinson's disease and anxiety. There are few randomized, controlled trials of the Alexander Technique, but what evidence there is does seem to point to its effectiveness, at least temporarily, in reducing pain and anxiety and improving breathing function in normal people.

In his evidence-based survey of complementary treatments,[24] Edzard Ernst cites several controlled trials (the "gold standard" of research) of normal, healthy subjects. These studies found that the Alexander Technique improved respiratory function,[25] chronic asthma,[26] and the ability of elderly women to reach for things.[27]

In uncontrolled trials (which do not use a control group for comparison), studies found that 67 people with chronic lower back pain reported improvements that persisted for six months after treatment in a multidisciplinary program that included lessons in the Alexander Technique.[28] In another "observational" study, seven patients with Parkinson's disease reported improvements in depression and the performance of daily activities.[29] Ernst also reports multiple cases of successes with the Alexander technique in people with craniomandibular (head and jaw) disorders.[30]

9

CRANIAL OSTEOPATHY AND CRANIOSACRAL THERAPY: MOVEMENT IS ALL

"Osteopaths focus on the structure of the body and how it functions," explains Rachel Brooks, M.D. "The goal is to restore the free, natural flow of movement at all levels, whether in the bones and joints, muscles and ligaments, the organs within their sheaths of connective tissue, or the flow of blood, lymph fluid or the cerebrospinal fluid that bathes and cushions the spinal cord and nerves throughout the body." Dr. Brooks lives in Portland, Oregon, and is a graduate of the University of Michigan Medical School. "Though an M.D. by training, I've devoted my whole professional life to osteopathy," she says.

Dr. Andrew Taylor Still, a physician who served

in the Union Army, founded osteopathy in the late 1800s. "After his wife and children died in an epidemic of spinal meningitis, Dr. Still became disillusioned with the tools of allopathic medicine," says Dr. Brooks. "He developed osteopathy as a hands-on way to treat people that built on what he believed to be the body's own inherent capacity to heal." Dr. Still developed a method of using the hands to affect the structure of the body to encourage and restore the free and natural flow of movement on every level.

Some of the key principles of osteopathy are:

- The body is a unit; the person is a unit of body, mind and spirit.
- The body is capable of self-regulation, self-healing and health maintenance.
- The structure and function of the whole body are related.

There are a number of manipulative approaches in osteopathy. Dr. Brooks practices a type called "cranial osteopathy," an extremely gentle practice that she uses to treat problems related to injury and illness. She can use the method to treat pain throughout the body resulting from muscle strain or trauma, infections and menstrual problems, as well as many other conditions.

Our bodies are never still, says Dr. Brooks. In addition to the beating of our hearts and the breath that flows in and out of our lungs, there is a constant pulse of movement throughout our organs and tissues. "Cranial osteopaths work from the principle that this constant, natural 'pulsing' within the body is how the body maintains itself in a state of health," she says, explaining that this pulsing has been linked to the slow, rhythmic movement of the cerebrospinal fluid originally described by osteopathic physician William Garner Sutherland in the 1930s. "By finding out where this rhythm is blocked, whether it is caused by injury or illness, and then helping the body to release that blockage, we can reduce pain and restore health," says Dr. Brooks. "For example, promoting a greater flow of lymph fluid, which helps to clear infection, allows the body to work more efficiently to recover from pneumonia and other infectious diseases."

How Cranial Osteopathy Works

"Many people think of the head as a solid 'bowling ball' type of structure, but that is not the case," says Dr. Brooks. "The bones of a newborn's skull are moveable and then become connected by seams, called sutures, as we grow. The skull solidifies, but even in the adult it always retains a resilience in the suture connections. I could train you to place your hands on someone's head and feel the slight, rhythmic, rocking movement that is normally present."

During a session of osteopathy, you lie fully clothed on a table; in some cases, the doctor may also have you sit or stand. Dr. Brooks explains that in every case she first examines the whole body to find out where the restrictions are, even if they are not located near the area of the symptoms. "Often, restrictions elsewhere in the body can have important effects on the area where the symptoms are," she explains. "I do not apply a significant force from the outside," she says. "I use my hands and my own intention to help the body find a state of balance and support it while allowing the tissues to release. I have found that adults with head or neck injuries and pain respond well to this treatment."

Over the years since Dr. Still created the practice of osteopathy, it has entered into the field of mainstream medicine. Doctors of osteopathy (D.O.) are certified to practice all medical specialties, including surgery. However, they also add a more holistic approach as well as their special training in osteopathic manipulation.

Craniosacral Therapy: Tapping Into the Wellspring of the Body

While general osteopathy and cranial osteopathy are performed by doctors of osteopathy, a similar treatment, called craniosacral therapy, can be performed by other practitioners, such as chiropractors, massage therapists, nurses and physical therapists. Craniosacral therapy grew out of the system of osteopathy and treats the central nervous system and its relationship to the spinal cord in a similar way. The craniosacral "rhythm" within the body comes from the regular pulsing of the liquid—called cerebrospinal fluid—that bathes, nourishes and protects the spinal cord. It is through the regular pulses of the cerebrospinal fluid that the brain transmits nerve messages to keep the body alive and functioning. No matter who the practitioner is, the most important component in effective treatment is that the practitioner takes into account the condition of the entire body, and that neither of these techniques replace necessary conventional treatment.

Dr. Eurydice Hirsey is one such practitioner, a chiropractor who is also trained in craniosacral therapy. "During a session, I begin to 'listen' to the craniosacral rhythm—which is much slower than a heartbeat, pulsing only six to twelve cycles per minute—by placing my hands on the sacrum (base of the spine), other areas of the spine and on the head, where I can feel the movement of the bones of the skull," says Dr. Hirsey. As Dr. Brooks pointed out, the head is actually made of separate, movable "bony plates" that are connected at seams or "sutures." "Through my hands, I feel the vitality, strength and symmetry of the craniosacral rhythm. I can also feel where there are restrictions to the flow of fluid throughout the body."

Blockages or restrictions in the craniosacral fluid can result from tension in the muscles or "fascia," the tissue just under the skin that overlies muscle and some organs, like a kind of inner "sleeve." These restrictions can be a response to physical or emotional trauma. "As I place my hands on the spine and head of my patient, I can often feel enormous resistance to the flow of cerebrospinal fluid, caused by blockages in the tissue," says Dr. Hirsey. "Any injury or trauma that alters or minimizes the flow of this fluid can cause pain and have a negative effect on our well-being and health."

During a session of craniosacral therapy, you lie on your back, fully clothed, on a cushioned table. As the practitioner places her hands under your back and on the connection between your head and neck, there is no sensation of "forcing" a movement. "I try to detect and focus on the deepest reservoir of the body, below the 'radar' of the conscious mind and even of the muscle," says Dr. Hirsey. "I often just follow the body's own impulse, gently helping it to undo the resistance in its own way, without pushing on the muscles or joints. This is how craniosacral work differs from chiropractic or even massage, where the practitioner might force or create a change in the body." It is the patient's own response to the practitioner's gentle touch that provides the release.

When the muscle resistance does finally relax, the sensation is one of deep release from a tension you might not have been aware of. "For some people this can be an enormous, sometimes volcanic release," said Dr. Hirsey. "They may cry, laugh or feel anger, often depending on whether the physical restriction in the body came from an emotional trauma."

Cranial Osteopathy: What's the Evidence?

Research on cranial osteopathy is not plentiful and needs to be broadened. Several studies show a benefit for children with asthma, recurrent ear infections,[31] developmental delays[32] and attention-deficit disorders.[33] In addition, some studies do indicate that it is effective for musculoskeletal pain,[34] especially for post-operative recovery and lower back pain, although one study found no significant difference between osteopathic treatment and standard medical care.[35]

Craniosacral Therapy: What's the Evidence?

No controlled trials of craniosacral therapy seem to exist, according to Dr. Edzard Ernst, who surveyed the literature and points out that Dr. Upledger himself, who developed the technique, does not cite them in his own writing. "Even though small movements between cranial bones are possible, there is no good evidence to suggest that restrictions of these movements have any health-related relevance," writes Dr. Ernst.[36]

However, practitioners, patients and parents claim that the technique is beneficial for problems such as birth trauma, chronic pain, cerebral dysfunction, cerebral palsy, colic, depression, dyslexia, ear infections, headaches, learning disabilities, Ménière's disease, musculoskeletal problems, migraine, sinusitis and stroke. Young children are believed to respond particularly well.

10

CHIROPRACTIC

The word "chiropractic" comes from the ancient Greek *cheiro* ("hand") and *praktikos* ("doing"). Chiropractors use their hands, as well as diagnostic tests and x-rays, to diagnose and treat disorders or misalignment of the spine. Distortions of the spine are thought to interrupt or damage messages that the brain sends through the central nervous system (the main branch of which is housed in the spine) to the rest of the body.

In her work as a chiropractor, Dr. Eurydice Hirsey, whom you met in the last chapter, treats patients with problems that include headaches and back, neck, shoulder, arm and leg pain. "Chiropractic is based on the premise that pain and a sense of malaise or 'dis-ease' (lack of ease) in the body come from a dysfunction in the spine, affecting both the central nervous system and the peripheral nervous system," says Dr. Hirsey. "The point of chiropractic is to get to the cause—where the nerves exit the spinal column, because distortions in these nerve messages can create problems throughout the body, affecting muscles, sensations, joints and organ systems."

The treatment involves orthopedic and neurological exams, as well as palpating (feeling) the muscles and joints to decide if there is a misalignment or malposition in the joints, vertebrae or pelvis. Chiropractors then use their hands in a technique called an "adjustment" to realign the vertebrae of the spine and the large joints of the body. (They also use a variety of other alignment methods.)

WHO SHOULD USE CHIROPRACTIC AND WHO SHOULDN'T?

Chiropractic can be used if you have musculoskeletal pain, but with the following cautions: For young children, make sure the therapist is trained in pediatric care. If you are over fifty, be cautious of neck manipulation because of the possibility of undiagnosed carotid artery disease and the related danger of stroke. If you have a connective disorder such as Marfan's syndrome or Ehlers-Danlos syndrome, or if you have had a spinal fusion or a tumor of the spine, you should not have chiropractic manipulations.

Chiropractic: What's the Evidence?

Research on chiropractic is generally considered inadequate, but the evidence is growing according to two summary reviews. "Historically, chiropractic has not had an adequate basis in scientific and academic research; it has not attained adequate research funding from government or the public sector," writes Kenneth Pelletier, Ph.D., M.D., (hon) former director of the Complementary and Alternative Medicine Program at Stanford University School of Medicine. "However, there are more than fifty RCTs (randomized controlled trials) in the chiropractic research literature, and the scientific basis for chiropractic is growing steadily."[37]

One of these studies is particularly noteworthy, according to Dr. Pelletier. In an evaluation of twenty-five controlled clinical trials, "there was a 17 percent greater likelihood of recovery from uncomplicated, acute low back pain within three weeks than without it."[38] And in a single long-term study of 741 patients, chiropractic was compared to hospital outpatient management for low back pain. "After three years, the chiropractic group had improved 29 percent more than the hospital group," summarizes Pelletier.[39]

A second overall review of the literature is less encouraging. The basic premise of chiropractic, which is that malalignment (subluxation) of the vertebrae causes disease, "has no scientific rationale," writes Edzard Ernst, M.D., Ph.D., F.R.C.P. (Edin), professor of complementary medicine and director of the Department of Complementary Medicine at the School of Postgraduate Medicine and Health Sciences, University of Exeter (United Kingdom). One systematic review by a chiropractor suggests that "there is moderate evidence of short-term efficacy" in the treatment of acute low back pain when compared with placebo and commonly used therapies. For mixed chronic and acute back pain, and for sciatica, the evidence was inconclusive. Ernst also highlights two other recent trials that did not demonstrate a convincing benefit of chiropractic over other forms of routine lower back pain treatments. "The bottom line of this somewhat confusing situation," suggests Ernst, "is that the effectiveness of chiropractic treatment of back pain is uncertain."[40]

And here is Dr. Pelletier's bottom line: "A small body of published clinical evidence now suggests that spinal manipulation may be helpful for fibromyalgia, high blood pressure, asthma, menstrual pain, infantile colic, otitis media, childhood enuresis (bedwetting), dizziness and vertigo, chronic pelvic pain, and other conditions."[41]

Lower Back and Pelvic Pain

A woman in her fifties, whom we will call Pamela, came to see chiropractor and craniosacral therapist Dr. Eurydice Hirsey for help with low back and pelvic pain that had become so severe it was creating problems with walking. After several sessions it became clear to Dr. Hirsey that this particular pain was originating from tightness in Pamela's stomach and abdomen. (But remember that this is only one possible cause of lower back pain.) "As I worked with Pamela, she began to talk about the horrible emotional abuse she had endured as a child," said Dr. Hirsey. "The safest way for her to deal with her anger and trauma was to hold it in check, and where she held it was in her stomach. Years of holding tension in her abdomen caused the muscles of her lower back and pelvis to remain chronically contracted, and the result was pain."

Slowly, over a period of months, Dr. Hirsey would place her hands gently on areas of tension in Pamela's body and "listen" for the pulsation of her craniosacral rhythm, deep in the spinal column. "I tried to guide her body to reduce its resistance to its own natural rhythm. Sometimes this would involve just waiting quietly. When Pamela's muscles relaxed, and the resistance melted away, I would often feel an actual motion or a sensation of warmth under my hand. If the release was dramatic, she might cry or report that she was reliving feelings of anger."

Pamela still comes to see Dr. Hirsey, but less often now. She has begun to breathe deeply from her abdomen, the way children do naturally, and has regained movement in her pelvis and lower back. Her pain has been significantly reduced and she has started yoga classes. "Breathing from her abdomen has helped bring more oxygen into her system," says Dr. Hirsey. "She reports that she feels happier now, more energetic. The physical release is helping her heal emotionally and spiritually, and she is continuing this work in psychotherapy."

When she is able to help patients like Pamela, Dr. Hirsey feels what she describes as total joy. "To be the most complete person, you have to be a member of the world and do what you can to help others. I want people to be out of pain, to walk again, to be whole, and then to help make the world whole." she says. "The most important thing is love for ourselves and those around us. If you can heal yourself, you can heal the world." Not surprisingly, Dr. Hirsey's business cards, decorated with colorful drawings by Nicaraguan artists, bear the slogan "Healing for Peace."

Herbal Treatments for Lower Back Pain

Always use herbs in consultation with your doctor and a certified herbalist.

- Bromelain with rutin and trypsin (Phlogenzym)
- Calcium
- Grape seed
- Magnesium
- Omega-3
- PA-free petasites (Butterbur)
- Pine bark
- Quercetin
- SAM-e
- Teasel
- Vitamin C (prevents disc degeneration)

11

AYURVEDIC MEDICINE

For Geeta, fibromyalgia meant a twenty-year struggle with pain. She felt exhausted all the time. "I had hardly any energy, but at the same time had difficulty sleeping," she says. "I had pain in my whole body and felt, at varying times, cold, dizzy and anxious. I had chronic sinus infections and allergies and a feeling that was close to hypoglycemia (when the blood sugar is low)."

Despite extensive testing, her conventional doctors could not diagnose her problem, although they did prescribe medications for the pain and insomnia. "I also tried acupuncture, Chinese herbal medicine and homeopathy, but nothing helped," says Geeta. "I did some research on my own and realized that I was suffering from fibromyalgia.

A native of India, Geeta decided to explore Ayurvedic medicine, the ancient medical system of India. "Ayurvedic medicine is something that most people in India know automatically, because we grow up using the herbs and natural remedies in our homes," says Geeta. "My mother would give us turmeric powder and honey in hot milk for any internal injury or infections. If we had muscle or joint pain, we would make a 'dough' of turmeric powder, whole wheat flour, and a little salt, heat it in a flat pan, wrap it in a cloth and apply it as a poultice to the affected area to speed healing. Turmeric powder is used for minor cuts because it has a kind of 'antiseptic' property."

For skin problems, including eczema, pimples and dermatitis, Geeta remembers garlic—lots of it. "My mother would serve us a clove of garlic with meals and crush fresh garlic to put on our skin. This would heal the problem," she says. "And always, during cold weather, we would have extra ginger in our food, as well as ginger powder in hot milk. It helps to keep the whole body system warm."

One of Geeta's best memories (one that might sound particularly wonderful to Westerners) involves the people who came to the houses in her neighborhood each week to give Ayurvedic massages to everyone in the family. "The Ayurvedic belief is that the whole body needs to be massaged regularly with certain oils to help keep the mind grounded in the body. When someone massages your whole body, it helps to integrate and connect your mind with your body. And besides, it felt absolutely wonderful!"

TIPS FROM AYURVEDIC MEDICINE

- Stir turmeric powder and honey in hot milk for internal injuries, stomach upset and infections.
- Make a "dough" of turmeric powder, whole wheat flour and a little salt, heat it in a flat pan, wrap it in a cloth and apply it as a poultice to areas of muscle or joint pain to speed healing.
- Use turmeric powder on minor cuts for its antiseptic and healing properties.
- Rub crushed garlic on the skin for eczema, pimples and dermatitis.
- Use extra ginger on food and ginger powder in hot milk to keep the whole body system warm during cold weather.
- Massage with warmed oils for pain and general well-being.

Geeta decided to work with an Ayurvedic practitioner, who helped her establish and stick to a
daily routine that included regular exercise and
meditation, yoga and deep breathing exercises. She
also received regular Ayurvedic massages with
warm essential oils. Ayurvedic practitioners ana-
lyze their patients' individual body types—called
"doshas"—and emotional makeup, and also prescribe certain foods and herbs that help to correct
imbalances. Based on her individual body type,
Geeta's practitioner advised her to eliminate red
meat, but eat plenty of stews with cooked vegetables, soups, cooked grains and other warm, com-
forting foods. She needed calming and warming
food—along with certain herbs—in order to
reduce the imbalance that was producing anxiety,
insomnia, muscle tension and other symptoms.
(Other people might receive different advice.)

Over a period of several months, Geeta noticed
improvements in her health and general outlook on
life for the first time in twenty years. "The massages
and yoga caused the pain to lessen, the breathing
and meditation calmed my mind and lowered the
level of anxiety, and my energy level came up with
the dietary changes and herbs. I am sleeping better
and have a more positive outlook on life. Now, the

only time I have pain is when I am under stress, but even then it doesn't last that long."

Ayurvedic Doshas—Body Types

Ayurvedic medicine classifies people into three basic "doshas" or body types, although most people may have characteristics of two or even three of the doshas.

Vata

Vata represents the elements of air and space. Vata people tend to be active, changeable and energetic. They are usually tall and slender. They can be anxious, unpredictable, alert and restless. When they are out of balance, vata people are prone to conditions that include nervous system problems, insomnia, arthritis, sciatica, lower back pain, constipation or intestinal gas. Vata people need food choices as well as herbs, meditation and breathing exercises, to help them stay calm.

Pitta

Pitta represents the elements of fire and water. Pitta people represent transformational energy. They are aggressive, explosive and efficient. When their energy is out of balance, pitta people are likely to have liver and gallbladder problems, gastritis, hyperacidity, peptic ulcer, inflammatory disease, and skin problems, including hives and acne. They should avoid hot, spicy foods, citrus fruit and excess sun exposure.

Kapha

Kapha represents the union of earth and water. Kapha is the densest of the three qualities. Kapha people tend to be slow-moving, conservative, stable and sometimes overweight. They can also be tranquil, stubborn and procrastinating. They tend to have slow digestion, a strong appetite and enjoy easy, deep sleep. When their energy is out of balance, kapha people tend to suffer from bronchitis, sinusitis, tonsillitis and lung congestion. They should avoid cheese, milk, yogurt, ice cream and cold drinks. In addition to respiratory problems, kapha people are also prone to allergies and gallstones.

Yoga

Developed in India over five thousand years ago, yoga[42] is a comprehensive, time-tested system of personal development. Yoga is not a religion; rather, it is a spiritual path that is complementary to all religions. The word "yoga" comes from a Sanskrit root that means "joining." The practice of yoga joins together body and mind, conscious self and inner self, and the individual spirit with a universal consciousness, which some call "the divine."

There are many kinds of yoga, but many Americans are most familiar with the physical exercises called "hatha" yoga, a meditative mind/body practice that involves physical postures called "asanas," breathing exercises called "pranayama" and deep relaxation. The postures stretch and tone the muscles and joints, the breathing exercises release tension as well as energy, and the relaxation practices bring body, mind and spirit back into their natural state of balance and wholeness.

Research has found that the physical postures, breathing and relaxation that make up a complete hatha yoga practice have powerful health-promoting effects, including lowering blood pressure and reducing the body's stress response, alleviating depression, and enhancing both self-awareness and the body's ability to heal itself. Studies have shown that yoga's physiological benefits include increasing strength and flexibility, improving endurance and helping to treat heart disease, chronic pain, asthma and digestion problems, among many other illnesses.

When many people think of yoga, exotic postures come to mind. In reality, though, yoga is not so much about twisting yourself into a pretzel or standing on your head, but more about learning how to stand firmly on your own two feet, in your body and in this moment. Through practicing hatha yoga, we learn to see beyond apparent opposites. The union of opposites and the balance of effort and surrender are reflected in the word "hatha" itself; "ha" means "sun" and "tha" means "moon."

Yoga quiets down the mind so we can experience peace and rediscover the unconditional happiness that lies beneath our mental "chatter." It also helps us to cultivate an inward focus, a greater awareness of our thoughts and feelings, and a stronger connection to our own healing presence. This connection enhances healing and creates the potential for spiritual awakening and transformation on physical, mental and emotional levels.

For information about how to find a yoga teacher and research about the health benefits of yoga, see Resources at the end of this book.

Headache and Migraine

When serious causes of head pain are ruled out, sometimes what is diagnosed as either tension headaches or migraines is the result of chronic tight muscles in the head and neck. These tight muscles may be the result of physical or emotional trauma, or anything that causes stress on the nervous system.

In general, you should keep your bowels moving, experiment with increasing or decreasing coffee, and avoid triggers such as specific foods, flickering lights and allergens. Here are some other steps you can take for tension or migraine headaches:

- *Proper hydration.* Drink seven or eight glasses of water daily. Room temperature is best.
- *Regular wake/sleep cycles.* Use herbs, yoga, meditation or whatever helps you wind down and relax at night. This encourages your brain to produce melatonin, which helps you sleep.
- *Craniosacral therapy or osteopathic manipulation therapy* may help.
- *Magnesium supplements (in the form of glycinate, gluconate, aspartate, oxide).* This is a natural

muscle relaxant and pain reliever and works particularly well for menstrual migraines. The recommended dosage, always in consultation with your doctor, is 250 to 500 milligrams orally twice a day. Note that this may cause diarrhea.

- *Riboflavin (Vitamin B2).* Take 200 milligrams twice a day for prevention of migraine in consultation with your doctor.
- *Massage therapy.*
- *Breathing and relaxation techniques, with guided imagery.*
- *Biofeedback.*
- *Acupuncture/acupressure.*
- *Herbal footbaths or compresses.* Use warm or cold baths, or even alternate using the calming herbs listed below.
- *Botanicals.* The following are recommendations from Dale Bellisfield, R.N., A.H.G. Always consult with your doctor. Those marked with an asterisk (*) taste good as teas.
  — **Migraines:** black cohosh, Chinese white peony, feverfew, ginger, PA-free petasites (butterbur).
  — **Constrictive "vicelike" headaches:** clematis, ginkgo.
  — **Dilative "your head feels like it is going**

to explode" headaches: feverfew, holy basil, lavender, rosemary.

— Hormonal headaches: cyperus, motherwort, vitex.

— Stress headaches: *chamomile, hops, kava, *lavender, *lemon balm, *meadowsweet, motherwort, *passionflower, *rosemary, valerian, *willow.

How to Use Ginger to Treat Migraine

Use ginger in capsules, tea or extracts. Ginger opens small blood vessels, has anti-inflammatory effects and relieves nausea (which often accompanies migraines). Take three to four times a day orally following package dosing instructions. Use caution if you are taking an anticoagulant as ginger thins the blood.

How to Use Feverfew to Prevent Migraines

Take feverfew as an extract or capsules. The typical dose is 50 to 100 milligrams, but follow package dosing instructions in consultation with your doctor. Use a whole-herb product.

Calming and Sedating Herbs

If your sleep habits are contributing to tension headaches, certified herbalist Dale Bellisfield, R.N., A.H.G., recommends that you consult with your doctor and a certified herbalist about the following herbs to help you wind down at the end of the day and have a restorative sleep. Those herbs marked by an asterisk (*) taste good as teas.

Blue vervain	*Lemon Balm
California poppy	*Linden
*Chamomile	Motherwort
*Fresh oat extract	Passionflower
Gambir	Scullcap
Hops	Valerian
*Lavender	Wood betony

12

MASSAGE THERAPY

Massage involves touch and movement. It is "the systematic manipulation of the soft tissues of the body to enhance health and healing," according to Lynda W. Freeman, Ph.D. Freeman summarizes the highlights of the massage therapy movement in the United States:

> In the nineteenth century, two physicians and brothers brought the "Swedish Movement Cure" to the United States, using their techniques to stimulate skin, muscle, blood vessels, the lymph system, nerves and some internal organs. The first massage therapy clinics in the United States were opened by the Swedes after the Civil War.

During the first part of the twentieth century, Swedish massage became popular at private health clubs and hospitals and with professional sports teams. The practice declined during the 1940s and '50s, coming back into prominence during the holistic health and healing movements of the '60s and '70s.[43]

Freeman credits a researcher's determination to help her own infant with the beginning of therapeutic massage—also known as touch therapy—as a medical treatment in this country. With the birth of her premature daughter, Tiffany Field, Ph.D., looked for ways to help her thrive and gain weight. "She massaged her daughter daily and found that this practice reduced the infant's anxiety, encouraged her to take more formula and helped her gain the weight. This led Dr. Field to hypothesize that similar and additional improvements might be observed in other premature infants if they were massaged in a similar manner."[44]

Dr. Field tested her hypothesis in several clinical trials, finding that premature infants who were massaged grew and developed better than those who were not massaged. She has since gone on to perform massage therapy research for other conditions and is now director of the Touch Research Institute at the University of Miami School of Medicine. Of course, the practice of massage in this country was going on long before Dr. Field began her research.

Today, the American Nurses Association recognizes massage therapy as an official nursing subspecialty, and therapeutic touch, an energy form of healing, was warmly embraced by nursing professionals. Of greater impact is the growing number of massage therapists performing full-time massage and body work. In some European countries, such as Germany, massage is considered part of conventional medicine.

This chapter highlights just two of the many types of massage therapy available.

Muscular Therapy: Melting Away Pain

When massage therapist Cindy Stewart presses on a muscle that is in spasm with just the right amount of pressure, she can actually feel it give way. "It is as if the hard muscle melts under my fingers," she says. "Muscles go into spasm for a good reason: usually to protect an injured ligament by restricting any motion that might cause further damage. But after the ligament heals, that tight muscle can create chronic pain."

Tight muscles are only one cause of pain. Scar tissue is another. "When ligaments or muscles are injured, even by tiny 'microtears,' scar tissue begins to form in six to eight days to repair the damage," Cindy explains. "Normally, this scar tissue—made of collagen—gets laid down over the injury like a tangled jumble of spaghetti, going in all directions. Often, this tangled collagen restricts the length-wise movement of the tissue, so people experience pain when they try to regain their full range of motion."

Most of Cindy's clients come to her because of chronic pain in the lower back and neck, usually caused by motor vehicle accidents or some other physical trauma. Their pain has restricted their lives. It affects the way they walk, what activities they can do and how they move their bodies in daily activity. They don't want to live on pain medications for the rest of their lives, so they turn to massage.

Cindy uses what she calls a "fractioning" technique to break up the tangled mass of collagen scar tissue that restricts movement and causes pain. The technique involves using her fingers to probe deeply into the area of the pain. "I use my fingers to massage across the width of the injured ligament, rather than the length," says Cindy. "This is called cross-fiber fractioning. By going *across* the ligament, I can begin to break up the collagen fibers of the scar tissue and encourage the body to lay down new *lengthwise* collagen that follows the line of the ligament and will not restrict movement." If this work is begun within a few days after the injury—within pain tolerance—you can often avoid the buildup of restrictive scar tissue in the first place.

Cindy describes one client who had such severe neck pain after a car accident that she could not turn her head. She also had some numbness in her arm. "She had tried physical therapy, but it did not give her permanent relief," says Cindy. "And she didn't want to do these exercises for the rest of her life." Cindy used the fractioning technique to break up the restrictive scar tissue, and she also gave her client "homework" that included icing the area and stretching exercises to keep the new scar tissue long and supple. After several weeks, the client regained more range of motion and the numbness disappeared. As an added bonus, her longstanding headaches became less intense and less frequent.

In addition to reducing scar tissue, the fractioning technique also works on tight muscles. "Because muscles cover a larger area, I might use all my fingers, or even my elbow, to go across the muscle and break up the tight fibers," explains Cindy. "By contrast, breaking up scar tissue on a ligament might take just one finger fractioning across the fibers."

No matter what part of the body Cindy is working on, she describes an almost "instinctive" feeling that guides her. "You need just the right amount of pressure to break up scar tissue, working within the client's pain tolerance; and if a muscle is in spasm, too much pressure might make it worse. You need to coax it to release," she says. "After so many years, I have learned to trust what I feel is going on under my fingers."

Oriental Bodywork Therapy: Tending the Garden

The first thing you see when you walk into Adele Strauss's waiting room is the almost full-size tiger under the coffee table. It is a very large toy, of course, but artistically constructed and almost startling in its realism. "He comes alive at night," says Adele with a smile. And indeed he looks like he might. He sits in regal repose, paws crossed, head held high, benignly surveying his small kingdom. He seems to fit in perfectly among the Chinese rosewood furniture, some of it antique, and the Oriental tapestry designs on the wall coverings and upholstery.

Adele began her study of bodywork with Oriental massage techniques. "Shiatsu is a Japanese massage method based on the principles of Chinese medicine," says Adele. "It is designed to move Qi energy that is stagnant by pressing with the hands on specific points on the body that lie along the energy pathways or meridians. I combine that pressure with stretching muscles, ligaments, sinews and tendons. This combination of pressure and stretching helps to move the 'stuck' Qi and restores the flow of vital energy in the body."

Over time, Adele began to combine shiatsu massage with *tui na*—a Chinese deep tissue massage that incorporates similar pressure and stretching techniques along the energy pathways of the body. "I developed my own combination of massage techniques that I call 'Oriental bodywork therapy,'" says Adele. "I feel like a gardener, tending the bodies of my patients, strengthening their vital energy so that they can begin to heal themselves." Nine years ago, Adele added acupuncture and herbal medicine to her "gardening" tools. She uses her combination of methods to treat conditions that include chronic pain, allergies, upper respiratory weakness and infections, chronic bronchitis, sinusitis, lung disorders, migraines, and gastrointestinal problems. "When my clients become discouraged, I sometimes say to them, 'You are not to blame for your pain or illness. For years, your body has responded to stress by tensing the muscles and secreting the fight-or-flight hormones. These responses are only meant to happen for a few moments, when, for example, a tiger is chasing you. But when it happens every day, over a period of years, it may cause chronic pain.'"

Massage: What's the Evidence?

I am the principal investigator of one of the first randomized, controlled clinical trials evaluating the effects of massage on osteoarthritis of the knee, involving sixty-four patients (in preparation for publication). My research suggests that massage therapy is an effective treatment to relieve pain and improve function in people with osteoarthritis of the knee.

One of the first researchers to test the benefits of massage, Dr. Tiffany Field found that "premature newborns who received massage therapy showed greater growth, weight gain and improved cognitive and motor development at eight months than non-massaged infants."[45] Since that time, research from randomized, controlled studies reviewed by Dr. Edzard Ernst suggests positive effects for anxiety, premenstrual syndrome and elderly institutionalized patients. For patients with fibromyalgia, it has been suggested to relieve pain and depression and improve the quality of life. It also was found to have potential for the treatment of both low back pain and chronic constipation.[46]

In her own review of the literature, Lynda W. Freeman, Ph.D., cites several studies finding that massage benefits not only patients with fibromyalgia, premenstrual and low back pain, as described above, but is also effective for other kinds of pain.[47] These include:

- *Cancer:* Male (but not female) cancer patients experienced significant short-term pain relief immediately after massage. Cancer patients also experienced increased mental clarity, general feelings of well-being, the release of unexpressed emotions and decreases in anxiety as a result of massage.
- *Surgical pain:* Patients admitted for abdominal

surgery were matched with a control group. The massaged group had significantly lower perceptions of pain in the twenty-four hours after surgery. Patients forty-one to sixty years old benefited the most.

- *Arthritis pain:* Children with juvenile rheumatoid arthritis (one of the most common chronic diseases of childhood) were massaged by their parents for fifteen minutes each night. Another group practiced relaxation with their parents for the same amount of time. At the end of thirty days, both the parents and children in the massage group experienced lower anxiety (determined by behavioral observation and levels of cortisol, a stress hormone, in the saliva). The massaged children reported significantly less pain after massage and fewer pain episodes than the relaxation group.

- *Migraine:* Massage therapy decreased the number of migraine headaches and reduced sleep disturbances and related distress symptoms.

- *Labor pain:* Women recruited from prenatal classes were assigned to massage in addition to Lamaze training. A control group had only Lamaze training. Laboring women received massage during the first fifteen minutes of each hour of childbirth. The massage group had less anxiety and pain, less need for medication, a significantly shorter labor period, a shorter hospital stay, and less post-partum depression than the control group.

- *Burn pain:* Massage therapy for burn patients reduced anxiety, anger, depression, pain and itching.

13

THE TRAGER® APPROACH:
EASING MIND AND BODY

The woman was in her mid-thirties, and no one could explain the constant, excruciating pain emanating from her lower back. She had seen doctors and tried many alternative treatments, all of which gave her only temporary relief. Her physician had finally referred her to Martin R. Anderson, a Trager practitioner.

"My colleague brought her to see me," remembers Martin. "She could barely walk into the office. She was hysterical, crying, and she said she was going to vomit. I had been practicing for nearly seventeen years, but at that moment my professional confidence nearly dropped to the floor. How could I possibly help her?"

Trager movement education, developed by the late Milton Trager, M.D., is an approach to the body that encourages mental and physical release, along with a feeling of openness, spaciousness and ease within the body. Practitioners learn to "hook-up" with the client, who lies fully clothed on a padded, comfortable table. Hooking up, Martin explains, brings him into an almost meditative state. "I try to connect—with compassion and understanding—with what the client is feeling at that moment, and to allow *her* to direct what I do next." During a typical session, Martin rhythmically moves the client's arms, legs and trunk with small, gentle rocking or "floppy" motions. At times he might also cradle the head, trying to sense where there might be potential release of tension. "While I work, I ask the client to tell me her response to the movements: Does this feel tighter? Looser? More or less painful?" says Martin. "At the same time I try to project a feeling of peace and calmness from deep within myself."

A typical session begins away from the table, with playful mental gymnastics, which Trager called Mentastics®. First, the practitioner asks, "What does this movement feel like? Is there a softness, an ease, an openness in your shoulder or hip?" When the client is ready, the work continues on the table. The next step is a deepening of the positive feeling: "Could it feel even lighter? Don't force it; just notice the feeling and see how your body answers." At this point, the practitioner might suggest a gentle modification of the movement and ask the client to notice the result. "Trager is an exploration," says Martin. "I might take a limb and play with it, move it in a different way, explore a new feeling of release. We do not 'work' tight muscles; we try to project a sense of lightness. The idea behind the practice is to help nerves send new messages to the brain —messages that communicate pathways to ease and freedom of movement, rather than the messages of tightness and pain that might have become a habit. Milton Trager used to say, 'There are no tight muscles, only tight minds.'"

When faced with his sobbing patient, Martin needed to look very deep within himself. "I got into a meditative state as I helped her get onto the table and propped her up with pillows," he says. "I then started a very gentle, rocking motion of her legs, not going anywhere near the painful back area, trying to send messages of peaceful, quiet movement to her back from my own mind and from the leg motions. I kept talking with her the whole time, asking, 'Does this movement feel okay? How about this?'"

The woman began to relax, even taking a few deep breaths. "Every time she took a breath, I would say, 'That looks like a lovely, deep breath.' Eventually, she stopped crying. Then I came up to her head and did a gentle massage of her temples, face and jaw; her breathing slowed and her body began to release tension. She said, 'You have very healing hands. I feel safe.' When that starts to happen, when the guard is let down, I can begin to send subtle messages of a new way of being in the body, trying to get around the fortress that was keeping her muscles so tight. I did a little rocking of the belly, then back to the legs."

After two hours, the woman got up from the table. "Before she did, I showed her a small lower back movement that she could do by herself at home to relieve pain," says Martin. "When she stood up, she said she had no pain for the first time in weeks, but she was afraid to move. Then she walked across the room and burst into tears because she felt no pain. I said to her, 'Your body knows how to organize itself like this, to move without pain and with deep relaxation. It came from your mind, and you can do it again. When you feel pain coming on, remember how it felt to be on this table.' Milton Trager called this phenomenon 'recall.' Other people call it 'kinesthetic hypnosis.' But whatever we call it, I know that the only thing I did was help her gain access to the deeper part of her mind that was causing the holding of tension in the muscles.

"The no-pain situation lasted for a day and a half," says Martin. "Then it started to come back, but not so intensely. My colleague is still treating her with the Trager Approach, and the pain is becoming more manageable. She is not using any medication to control it."

Martin points out that the rhythmic Trager motions have helped several of his clients with diseases that induce muscle spasticity, including Parkinson's, multiple sclerosis and cerebral palsy. "When used along with conventional drugs and medical treatment, Trager can offer patients a balancing rhythm that counteracts the tremors and spastic movements," he says. "For example, I used the technique with a forty-five-year-old man, a psychiatrist, with severe Parkinson's; he had uncontrollable swinging motions of his arms. I got him on the table, and the rocking rhythm of my hands counteracted the spasticity, at least temporarily. He got off the table, his swinging motions stopped, and he said, 'I don't get it. It's too simple.'"

At the end of his life, when he was in his eighties, Milton Trager himself suffered from severe Parkinson's disease. Martin attended one of the last classes that he ever gave. "Word had it that he was very depressed and not well," says Martin. "So we were astonished when the classroom door flew open and in came Milton with his wife, Emily. He was holding a tape of Herb Alpert and the Tijuana Brass Band and insisted that we play it. He had discovered that strong musical rhythms helped to counteract his own tremors and spasticity. So we all danced around to the music, led by Milton, finding his own inner rhythm."

(For more information: *www.trager.com*)

14

MEDITATION: DON'T MISS A MOMENT OF YOUR LIFE

There are so many different kinds of meditation that sorting them out can be confusing. In *Essentials of Complementary Medicine*, Lynda Freeman has a useful way of looking at the variations, which she divides into two basic forms: concentrative meditation and open meditation. Within each of these forms there are many types.

Concentrative Meditation

In concentrative meditation forms, you focus your attention on one stimulus—a word or phrase, an object such as a candle, or your breath. If your attention strays, you gently bring it back to focus on the stimulus, over and over again. This form of meditation produces a "disciplined mind that can be still and at peace," with health benefits that include interrupting "repetitive and negative thought patterns that feed anxiety and depression. . . . "[48]

Types of concentrative meditation include:

- Transcendental Meditation, founded by Maharishi Mahesh Yogi
- Formal Buddhist sitting meditation
- The "Respiratory One Method" (ROM) developed by Herbert Benson, M.D., who performed the original research on Transcendental Meditation and also developed the concept of the "relaxation response."

Open Meditation

In open meditation you don't try to restrict your attention to only one stimulus (which is the concentrative method). Instead, you observe your thoughts, your bodily sensations and the sounds around you. The idea is to observe without judging them as good or bad, detaching your emotions and lowering your "reactivity" to what is going on. The goal is for negative thoughts and emotions to "lose their grip" and their power over your well-being. The most widely used method of open meditation is "Vipassana," also called "mindfulness" or "awareness" meditation, which is based on Buddhist practices and was developed for clinical use by Jon Kabat-Zinn, Ph.D. "This form of meditation seeks to observe what the concentrative methods seek to ignore (i.e., everyday life events and experiences). . . . The final goal is a state of continual nonjudgmental observation—of being totally 'awake' to the world, enlivened by life events, not overwhelmed by them."[49]

Meditation When You Are in Pain

The essence of mindfulness meditation, according to meditation teacher Fern Ross Israel, is to develop a practice of awareness in everyday life, without the distractions of memories of the past (which is no longer here) or thoughts about the future (which has not yet arrived). This is most often done by focusing on the breathing; the movement of breath in and out of the body is a good way to remind yourself of the reality of the present moment. The benefit is freedom, calmness and inner peace. "You can bring this relaxed, centered presence to the chaos and ups and downs of life," says Fern. "When something happens, you don't have to react 'on automatic pilot.' You can stop, *see clearly* what is happening (instead of through the foggy lens of preconceived ideas), *reflect* calmly, and then *choose* how you will react, rather than allowing yourself to succumb to your habitual reaction patterns."

Among its other benefits, mindfulness is a very good way to deal with physical pain. "With practice, patients can learn to observe the changing nature of the pain and hold their experience with compassion," says Fern. "When I meditate with patients, we often refer to these sensations as 'the' pain or 'our' pain. This can change the experience of pain for some people, by allowing them to separate it from the essence of who they are." One of Fern's areas of expertise is working with seriously ill and dying patients and their families. One of her patients was a young woman with a rare cancer that spread quickly through the fatty tissue of her body, causing great pain and eventually killing her within six months. "I taught her meditation and worked with her during her treatment and later in hospice," says Fern. "Her mother told me that the meditation practice helped her daughter more with the pain than the morphine drip she was given in hospice care."

HOW TO MEDITATE: AN INTRODUCTION

The best recommendation is to find a meditation class in your community, but here is some guidance if you want to get started right away:

- Choose a quiet corner.
- Set a timer for five minutes.
- Sit with crossed legs on the floor on a cushion or on a chair.
- Keep your back very straight. You can use a chair with a back if needed. Imagine the top of your head is touching the sky.
- Put your hands palms up and open on your knees.
- Close your eyes.
- Breathe in and out slowly. You might want to count your breaths.
- Do not move at all except to keep your back straight.
- Name the things that come to your mind: "I feel bored," "My right knee hurts," then bring back your attention to your breathing.
- Pay attention to your sensations: breathing, aches, itches, fears. Let them happen.
- Stop when the timer rings.

Meditation: What's the Evidence?

The practice of meditation has been in use for thousands of years in many cultures, including Buddhist, Ayurvedic and Taoist traditions. Meditation

practices in various forms have shown health benefits: In clinically controlled trials, mindfulness or
awareness meditation has been demonstrated to
effectively reduce anxiety and depression, including the condition known as post-traumatic stress
disorder; to significantly reduce chronic pain
caused by a variety of medical conditions; to
increase life functionality; and to reduce mood dis-
turbance and psychiatric symptoms. Most of these
outcomes were achieved with patients who had
not improved with traditional medical care.[50]

In this country, there has been more than thirty
years of research into various meditation practices,
beginning with Herbert Benson, M.D., who performed the original research on the outcomes of
Transcendental Meditation (a form of concentration meditation founded by Maharishi Mahesh
Yogi). Dr. Benson is perhaps best known for developing and researching the "relaxation response."

Mindfulness Meditation for Anxiety and Chronic Pain

Jon Kabat-Zinn, Ph.D., founded the Stress
Reduction Clinic at the University of Massachusetts
Medical Center in 1979. He is credited with
adapting the Buddhist practice of Vipassana

meditation into "mindfulness meditation" for clinical use. This form of meditation is now used throughout the United States in hospital-based stress management programs.

Kabat-Zinn's clinical research in the Stress Reduction Program demonstrated the effectiveness of an outpatient group program based on mindfulness meditation in the treatment of anxiety. A follow-up study three years later "strongly suggests the long-term effectiveness" of the program, although he notes that both studies "lacked a randomized control group for comparison and a control for concomitant treatment."[51] In an earlier study, Kabat-Zinn demonstrated that a ten-week mindfulness meditation program was "an effective behavioral program in self-regulation for chronic pain patients."[52]

And You Don't Even Have to Be Sick

In addition to reducing pain, anxiety, depression and other symptoms of illness, Michael J. Baime reports that "meditation also benefits individuals without acute medical illness or stress. People who meditate regularly report that they feel more confidant and more in control of their lives. They say that their relationships with others are improved and that they experience more enjoyment and appreciation of life."[53]

Lynda Freeman argues forcefully for the inclusion of meditation in clinical practice: "In medicine, there is a tendency to 'standardize' a treatment, to strip that treatment of subjective as opposed to objective meaning, and to remove issues of consciousness from the outcome. If people have learned nothing else from consciousness and meditation research, it is that this approach is simplistic and ineffectual. Humans need to transform and grow just as they need food and water. . . . Consciousness and the need for transformation will not conform to medical opinion; medical thought is going to need to adapt to these critical issues of consciousness, as they relate to medical outcomes."[54]

RESOURCES

For details about complementary/alternative practices, including all those mentioned in this book, see R. Weisman and B. Berman, *Own Your Health: Choosing the Best from Alternative and Conventional Medicine*. HCI books 2003.

These organizations, Web sites and publications provide information on both conventional and complementary and alternative medicine (CAM) and research.

Alexander Technique

Alexander Technique International

Web site: *www.ati-net.com*

Alexander, F. M. *The Use of Self*. London: Gollancz, 1996.
An account of how Alexander developed the method.

Conable, Barbara. *How to Learn the Alexander Technique: A Manual for Students*. Andover Press, 1995.

Jones, Frank Pierce. *Body Awareness in Action: A Study of the Alexander Technique*. Schocken, 1987.

Biofeedback, Hypnotherapy, Guided Imagery for Pain

Academy for Guided Imagery

Web site: *www.healthy.net/agi*

Julietta Appleton, Certified Hynotherapist (interviewed for this book)
E-mail: *juliettaappleton@aol.com*

Association for Applied Psychophysiology and Biofeedback
Web site: *www.aapb.org*

Gary L. Goldberg, Health Psychologist (interviewed for
this book)
Phone: (973) 992-2888

Government Resources

CAM on PubMed
Web site: *www.nlm.nih.gov/nccam/camonpubmed.html*

This collection of more than 220,000 citations is accessed
through the PubMed database, which also includes
Medline.

ClinicalTrials.Gov
Web site: *www.clinicaltrials.gov*
ClinicalTrials.Gov provides a complete listing of all
CAM trials sponsored by the National Institutes of
Health. For a complete listing of clinical studies in
CAM, search under the key words "alternative medicine."

Combined Health Information Database (CHID)
Web site: *http://chid.nih.gov*
The federally supported Combined Health
Information Database (CHID) includes a variety of
materials not available in other government databases.
CHID aggregates health information for the public on
numerous topical areas related to health and disease.

The National Center for Complementary and Alternative
Medicine (NCCAM)
Web site: *http://nccam.nih.gov*
The NCCAM is dedicated to exploring complementary and alternative healing practices in the context of
rigorous science, training CAM researchers and dis-
seminating authoritative information to health care
consumers and patients. NCCAM funds and monitors
more CAM research than any other institution in the
United States.

The National Center for Complementary and Alternative
Medicine (NCCAM) Public Information
Clearinghouse
P.O. Box 7923
Gaithersburg, MD 20898
Phone: 1-888-644-6226; outside U.S.: (301) 519-3153
Fax: 1-866-464-3616 (Toll-Free)
TTY: 1-866-464-3615 (Toll-Free)
E-mail: *info@nccam.nih.gov*
Web site:
http://nccam.nih.gov/health/clearinghouse/index.htm
As one of its mandates from Congress, NCCAM is
charged with "the dissemination of health informa-
tion. In respect to identifying, investigating, and
validating complementary and alternative treatment,
diagnostic, and prevention modalities, disciplines, and
systems" (Public Law 105-277). The NCCAM
Clearinghouse serves this mission. It is the public's
point of contact for scientifically based information on
complementary and alternative medicine (CAM) and
for information about NCCAM.

Herbal Medicine and Dietary Supplements

American Botanical Council
Web site: *www.herbalgram.org*

American Dietetic Association
Web site: *www.eatright.org*

American Herbalists Guild
Web site: *www.americanherbalistsguild.com*

Dale Bellisfield, R.N., AHG, Certified Herbalist (interviewed for this book)
E-mail: *herbaldale@aol.com*

Natural Medicines Comprehensive Database
Web site: *www.naturalmedicines.com*

Natural Standards
  Web site: *www.naturalstandards.com*

Hypnotherapists Specializing in Fibromyalgia

Alabama Hypnotherapy Center and Hypnosis Associates
  Web site: *www.tranceworkers.com/fibromaplink.html*

Integrative Medicine

Carol and Morton Siegler Center for Integrative
  Medicine
  200 South Orange Avenue
  Livingston, NJ 07039
  Phone: (973) 322-7007
  Web site: *www.sbhcs.com/services/integrative/about-us.htm*

Institute for Complementary and Alternative Medicine
  University of Medicine and Dentistry of New Jersey
  Web site: *www.umdnj.edu/icam*

Fugh-Berman, Adrian. *Alternative Medicine: What Works:
  A Comprehensive, Easy-to-Read Review of the Scientific
  Evidence, Pro and Con.* William and Wilkins, 1997.

Rakel, David, ed. *Integrative Medicine.* W.B. Saunders
  Company, 2002.

Sarno, John E. *The Mindbody Prescription: Healing the
  Body, Healing the Pain.* Warner Books, 1999.

Massage

American Massage Therapy Association
  Web site: *www.amtamassage.org*

Herbalist & Alchemist (Essential Oils)
  Phone: (800) 611-8235

National Certification Board for Therapeutic Massage
  and Bodywork
  Web site: *www.ncbtmb.com*

Other Conventional and Complementary Resources

Acupuncture.com
   Web site: *www.acupuncture.com*

The Alternative Medicine Homepage
   Web site: *www.pitt.edu/~cbw/altm.html*

American Association of Oriental Medicine
   Web site: *www.aaom.org*

American Chiropractic Association
   Web site: *www.amerchiro.org*

American College of Rheumatology
   Web site: *www.rheumatology.org*

The Ayurvedic Institute
   Web site: *www.ayurveda.com*

HealthWorld Online (Mind/Body Resource Center)
   Web site: *www.healthy.net/cmbm*

National Certification Commission for Acupuncture and
   Oriental Medicine
   Web site: *www.nccaom.org*

Pain Management

American Chronic Pain Association
   P.O. Box 850
   Rocklin, CA 95677
   E-mail: ACPA@*pacbell.net*
   Web site: *www.theacpa.org*

American Pain Foundation
   111 South Calvert Street, Suite 2700
   Baltimore, MD, 21202
   Web site: *www.painfoundation.org*

Arthritis Foundation
   Web site: *www.arthritis.org*

Book: *The Arthritis Foundation's Guide to Alternative
   Therapies* by Judith Horstman, editor (1999).

Trager® Movement Education
Web site: *www.trager.com*

Yoga

The Yoga Site
Web site: *www.yogasite.com/articles.htm*
See article "Why Do Yoga?" at
www.yogasite.com/why.htm.
YogaFinder
Web site: *www.yogafinder.com*
A good site for finding a yoga teacher.
Yoga Alliance
Web site: *www.yogaalliance.org/index.php*
Yoga Alliance sets standards for and maintains a
registry of yoga teachers.

Yoga and Meditation Research

Bera, T., M. Gore and J. Oak. "Recovery from Stress in
Two Different Postures and in Shavasana—A Yogic
Relaxation Posture." *Indian J Physiol Pharmacol* 42(4)
(1998): 473–478.

Carrington, P. "The Physiology of Meditation." In: PM PL
and R. Woolfolk, eds. *Principles and Practice of Stress
Management*, 2nd ed. New York: Guilford, 1993, 141.

Corliss, R. "The Power of Yoga." *Time* 157: 54–62.

Davidson, R. "Alterations in Brain and Immune Function
Produced by Mindfulness Meditation." *Psychosom Med*
64(4) (2003): 564–570.

Jacobs, G. "The Physiology of Mind-Body Interactions:
The Stress Response and the Relaxation Response." *J
Altern Complement Med* 7(Suppl 1) (2001): S83–92.

Koertge, J., et al. "Improvement in Medical Risk Factors
and Quality of Life in Women and Men with
Coronary Artery Disease in the Multicenter Lifestyle

Demonstration Project." *Am J Cardiol* 91.11 (2003): 1316–1322.

Murugesan, R. N. Govindarajulu and T. Bera. "Effect of Selected Yogic Practices on the Management of Hypertension." *Indian J Physiol Pharmacol* 44(2) (2000): 207–210.

Raub, J. "Psychophysiologic Effects of Hatha Yoga on Musculoskeletal and Cardiopulmonary Function: A Literature Review." *J Alt Complementary Med* 8(6) (2002): 797–812.

Saraswati, S. S. *Yoga Nidra*, 6th ed. Bihar, India: Yoga Publications Trust, 1998.

Shannahoff-Khalsa, D. "An Introduction to Kundalini Yoga Meditation Techniques That Are Specific for the Treatment of Psychiatric Disorders." *J Altern Complement Med* 10(1) (2004): 91–101.

NOTES

1. Lynda W. Freeman, *Best Practices in Complementary and Alternative Medicine: An Evidence-Based Approach with Nursing CE/CME* (Gaithersburg, MD: Aspen Publishers, 2001), 3-1: 7.

2. Ester Shapiro, *Grief as a Family Process: A Cultural and Developmental Approach to Integrative Practice*, 2nd edition. New York, NY: Guilford, in press).

3. Ester Shapiro, "Chronic Illness as a Family Process," *Journal of Clinical Psychology*. 58:1375–1384, 2002.

4. James A. Duke, *The Green Pharmacy* (Emmaus, PA: Rodale, 1997), 55.

5. Sandra Blakeslee, "Complex and hidden brain in gut makes stomachaches and butterflies." *The New York Times*, 23 January 1996: 1.

6. James A. Duke, *The Green Pharmacy* (Emmaus, PA: Rodale, 1997), 283.

7. Ibid., 284.

8. For more details of all of his recommendations, see James A. Duke, *The Green Pharmacy*, (Emmaus, PA: Rodale, 1997).

9. John Sarno, *Mind Over Back Pain: A Radically New Approach to the Diagnosis and Treatment of Back Pain* (New York: Berkley Publishing Group, 1999); *www.healingbackpain.com/index2.html*.

10. Edzard Ernst, ed., *The Desktop Guide to Complementary and Alternative Medicine: An Evidence-Based Approach* (Edinburgh: Harcourt Publishers Limited, 2001), 41; and Sarno, *Mind Over Back Pain*.

11. Kenneth R. Pelletier, *The Best Alternative Medicine: What Works? What Does Not?* (New York: Simon & Schuster, 2000), 77.

12. Lixing Lao, "Traditional Chinese Medicine," in *Essentials of*

Complementary and Alternative Medicine, Wayne B. Jonas and Jeffrey S. Levin, eds. (Baltimore, MD, and Philadelphia, PA: Lippincott, Williams & Wilkins, 1999), 228.

13. G. B. Andersson, "Epidemiological Features of Chronic Low-Back Pain." *Lancet* 453 (1999): 581–585.

14. E. Manheimer et al., "Meta-Analysis: Acupuncture for Low Back Pain." *Ann Intern Med* 142 (2005): 651–663.

15. B. Berman et al., "Effectiveness of Acupuncture as Adjunctive Therapy in Osteoarthritis of the Knee: A Randomized Controlled Trial." *Ann Intern Med* 141 (2004): 901–910.

16. A.J. Vickers, "Can Acupuncture Have Specific Effects on Health? A Systematic Review of Acupuncture Antiemesis Trials." *J R Soc Med* 89(6) (1996): 303–311; J. W. Dundee et al., "The Role of Transcutaneous Electrical Stimulation of Neiguan Anti-Emetic Acupuncture Point in Controlling Sickness After Cancer Chemotherapy." *Physiotherapy* 77(7) (1991): 499–502.

17. B. M. Berman and J. P. Sawyers, "Complementary Medicine Treatments for Fibromyalgia Syndrome." *Baillieres Best Pract Res Clin Rheumatol* 13(3) (1999): 487–492; B. M. Berman et al., "Is Acupuncture Effective in the Treatment of Fibromyalgia?" *J Fam Pract* 48(3) (1999): 213–218; and L. Shoukang, "Treating Arthralgia with Acupuncture." *Internat J Clin Acup* 2(1) (1999): 71–76.

18. A. Richter et al., "Effect of Acupuncture in Patients with Angina Pectoris." *Eur Heart J* 12 (1991): 175–178.

19. D. Melchart et al., "Acupuncture for Idiopathic Headache." *Cochrane Database Syst Rev* (1) (2001): CD001218; and C.A. Vincent, "A Controlled Trial of the Treatment of Migraine by Acupuncture." *Clin J Pain* 5 (1989): 305–312.

20. M. A. Naeser et al., "Real Versus Sham Acupuncture in the Treatment of Paralysis in Acute Stroke Patients: A CT Scan Lesion Site Study." *J Neuro Rehab* 6 (1992): 163–173; K. Johanson et al., "Can Sensory Stimulation Improve the Functional Outcome in Stroke Patients?" *Neurology* 43 (1993): 2189–2192.

21. H. C. Haanen et al., "Controlled Trial of Hypnotherapy in the Ttreatment of Refractory Fibromyalgia." *J Rheumatol* 18(1) (1991): 72–75.

22. Albert Donnay and Grace Ziem, "Prevalence and Overlap of

Chronic Fatigue Syndrome and Fibromyalgia Syndrome Among 100 New Patients with Multiple Chemical Sensitivity." Copublished simultaneously in *Journal of Chronic Fatigue Syndrome* 5(3/4) (1999): 71–80; and in *Chronic Fatigue Syndrome: Advances in Epidemiologic, Clinical and Basic Science Research*, Roberto Patarca-Montero, ed., (Binghamton, NY: Haworth Medical Press, 1999), 71–80.

23. "Multiple Chemical Sensitivity: A Scientific Overview," U.S. Department of Health and Human Services: Public Health Service and Agency for Toxic Substances and Disease Registry, 1995.

24. Edzard Ernst, ed., *The Desktop Guide to Complementary and Alternative Medicine: An Evidence-Based Approach* (London, UK): Harcourt Publishers Limited, 2001).

25. J. H. M. Austin, et al., "Enhanced Respiratory Muscular Function in Normal Adults After Lessons in Proprioceptive Musculoskeletal Education Without Exercises." *Chest* 102 (1992): 486–490.

26. J. Dennis and C. Cates, "Alexander Technique for Chronic Asthma." *Cochrane Review* 2 (2002).

27. R. J. Dennis, "Functional Reach Improvement in Normal Older Women After Alexander Technique Instruction." *J Gerontol—Biol Sci Med Sci* 54 (1999): 8–11.

28. O. Elkayam et al., "Multidisciplinary Approach to Chronic Back Pain: Prognostic Elements of the Outcome." *Clin Exp Rheum* 14 (1996): 281–288.

29. C. Stallinbrass, "An Evaluation of the Alexander Technique for the Management of Disability in Parkinson's Disease—A Preliminary Study." *Clin Rehab* 11 (1997): 8–12.

30. S. Knebelman, "The Alexander Technique in Diagnosis and Treatment of Craniomandibular Disorders." *Basal Facts* 5 (1982): 19–22.

31. B. Gintis, "AAO Case Study. Recurrent Otitis Media." *AAOJ* 6(2) (1996): 16. (Cited in Jonas).

32. V. Frymann et al., "Effect of Osteopathic Medical Management on Neurologic Development in Children," *J Am Osteopath Assoc* 92 (1992): 729–744.

33. L. M. Agresti, "Attention Deficit Disorder. The Hyperactive Child." *Osteopathic Annals* 14 (1989): 6–16.

34. R. W. Jarski et al., "The Effectiveness of Osteopathic Manipulative Treatment as Complementary Therapy Following Surgery: A Prospective, Match-Controlled Outcome Study." *Altern Ther Health Med* 6(5) (2000): 77–81.

35. G. P. Andersson et al., "A Comparison of Osteopathic Spinal Manipulation with Standard Care for Patients with Low Back Pain." *N Engl J Med* 341(19) (1999): 1426–1431.

36. Edzard Ernst, ed., *The Desktop Guide to Complementary and Alternative Medicine: An Evidence-Based Approach* (Edinburgh: Harcourt Publishers Limited, 2001), 48.

37. Kenneth R. Pelletier, *The Best Alternative Medicine: What Works? What Does Not?* (New York: Simon & Schuster, 2000), 220.

38. Ibid. 221

39. Ibid. 221

40. Edzard Ernst, ed., *The Desktop Guide to Complementary and Alternative Medicine: An Evidence-Based Approach* (Edinburgh: Harcourt Publishers Limited, 2001), 46.

41. Kenneth R. Pelletier, *The Best Alternative Medicine: What Works? What Does Not?* (New York: Simon & Schuster, 2000), 224.

42. Yoga description courtesy of Matthew Fritts of the Samueli Institute.

43. Lynda W. Freeman, *Best Practices in Complementary and Alternative Medicine: An Evidence-Based Approach with Nursing CE/CME* (Gaithersburg, MD: Aspen Publishers, 2001), 3–1:2.

44. Ibid., 3–1:8.

45. T. Field et al., "Massage of Preterm Newborns to Improve Growth and Development." *Pediatric Nursing* 13 (1987): 385–387. (Cited in Freeman, *Best Practices in Complementary and Alternative Medicine.*)

46. Edzard Ernst, "Abdominal Massage Therapy for Chronic Constipation: A Systematic Review of Controlled Clinical Trials.," *Forsch Komplementarmed* 6 (1999): 149–151; and Edzard Ernst, Massage Therapy for Low Back Pain: A Systematic Review." *J Pain Symptom Manage* 17 (1999): 65–69.

47. Lynda W. Freeman, *Best Practices in Complementary and Alternative Medicine: An Evidence-Based Approach with Nursing CE/CME* (Gaithersburg, MD: Aspen Publishers, 2001), 3–1:4.

48. Ibid., 8–1:2

49. Ibid., 8–1:5.

50. Ibid., 8–1:1.

51. J. Kabat-Zinn, et. al. "Effectiveness of a Meditation-Based Stress Reduction Program in the Treatment of Anxiety Disorders." *American Journal of Psychiatry* 149 (1992): 9336–9943

    J. Kabat-Zinn, et. al. "Three-Year Follow-Up and Clinical Implications of a Mindfulness Meditation-Based Stress Reduction Intervention in the Treatment of Anxiety Disorders." *General Hospital Psychiatry* 17 (1995): 192–200.

52. J. Kabat-Zinn, "An Outpatient Program in Behavioral Medicine for Chronic Pain Patients Based on the Practice of Mindfulness Meditation," *General Hospital Psychiatry* 4 (1982): 33–47.

53. M. J. Baime and R. V. Baime, "Stress Management Using Mindfulness Meditation in a Primary Care General Internal Medical Practice," *J Gen Int Med* 11(S1) (1996): 131.

54. Lynda W. Freeman, *Best Practices in Complementary and Alternative Medicine: An Evidence-Based Approach with Nursing CE/CME* (Gaithersburg, MD: Aspen Publishers, 2001), 8-1:16.

ABOUT THE AUTHORS

Adam Perlman received his B.A. from Tufts University and his M.D. from Boston University School of Medicine. He completed residencies in both internal medicine and preventive medicine at Boston Medical Center, as well as a general medicine research fellowship and Masters of Public Health with a concentration in biostatistics and epidemiology from the Boston University School of Public Health.

He became director of Integrative Medicine for the Saint Barnabas Health Care System and Medical Director for the Carol and Morton Siegler Center for Integrative Medicine, in Livingston, New Jersey in 1998. In that role, he had primary responsibility for developing and overseeing the Complementary & Alternative Medicine Program, including both the Integrative Medicine Center and the Center for Health and Wellness for the largest healthcare system in New Jersey.

In 2002, Dr. Perlman became executive director for the Institute for Complementary and Alternative Medicine (ICAM) at the University of Medicine and Dentistry of New Jersey (UMDNJ), where he is an assistant professor of medicine. In 2004, he was named the UMDNJ Endowed Professor of Complementary and Alternative Medicine.

Roanne Weisman is an award-winning author specializing in science, medicine and health care. She is principal of Words That Work, a Massachusetts-based company that provides writing services to medical, academic and corporate clients. She has coauthored several books in the *Own Your Health* series.